HEALING
WITH
IODINE

YOUR MISSING LINK
TO BETTER HEALTH

D1595882

Other books by Dr. Mark Sircus

Anti-Inflammatory Oxygen Therapy

Healing with Medical Marijuana

Sodium Bicarbonate

HEALING WITH IODINE

YOUR MISSING LINK TO BETTER HEALTH

Dr. Mark Sircus

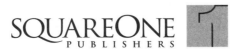

SQUAREONE
PUBLISHERS

COVER DESIGNER: Jeannie Tudor
EDITOR: Erica Shur
TYPESETTER: Gary A. Rosenberg

The information and advice contained in this book are based upon the research and the personal and professional experiences of the author. They are not intended as a substitute for consulting with a health care professional. The publisher and author are not responsible for any adverse effects or consequences resulting from the use of any of the suggestions, preparations, or procedures discussed in this book. All matters pertaining to your physical health should be supervised by a health care professional. It is a sign of wisdom, not cowardice, to seek a second or third opinion.

Square One Publishers
115 Herricks Road
Garden City Park, NY 11040
(516) 535-2010 ● (877) 900-BOOK
www.squareonepublishers.com

Library of Congress Cataloging-in-Publication Data

Names: Sircus, Mark, author.
Title: Healing with iodine : your missing link to better health / Dr. Mark Sircus.
Description: Garden City Park, NY : Square One Publishers, [2018] | Includes
    bibliographical references and index.
Identifiers: LCCN 2018007352 (print) | LCCN 2018007745 (ebook) | ISBN
    9780757054679 | ISBN 9780757004674
Subjects: LCSH: Iodine—Therapeutic use.
Classification: LCC RM666.I6 (ebook) | LCC RM666.I6 S57 2018 (print) | DDC
615.2734—dc23
LC record available at https://lccn.loc.gov/2018007352

Printed in the United States of America

10   9   8   7   6   5   4

Contents

*This book is dedicated to Dr. David Brownstein,
Dr. David Derry, Dr. Guy Abraham, Dr. Donald Miller Jr.,
and Dr. Tullio Simoncini for their courage of their
convictions in bringing back iodine as a universal medicine.*

Introduction

A recent article in the New York Times asked the question, "How important is iodized salt to the American or European diet?" The answer to the question was convoluted at best—deceiving at worst. "Most Americans who eat a varied diet get enough iodine even if they don't use iodized salt." Not true. Even if you add the iodized salt, it still would not be true.

According to the National Health and Nutrition Examination Survey, U.S. iodine levels have fallen nearly 50 percent over the last 40 years. Moreover, studies of women of childbearing age show that nearly 60 percent of U.S. women are deficient in iodine with over 10 percent severely deficient. In reality, the need for iodine has actually increased due to our constant exposure to halides—which are found in such common toxins as fluoride and bromide—that have increased in our environment. And according to the U.N.'s World Health Organization, iodine deficiency affects 72 percent of the world's population.

The New York Times acknowledged, "…some pregnant women are at risk of low iodine levels, which potentially endanger their babies." The use of the word "some" in that line is an understatement when you consider that 60 percent of women who are at an age for pregnancy are deficient in iodine.

Dr. David Brownstein and his partners have checked iodine levels on over 6,000 patients in the Detroit area, and the vast majority—over 97 percent—are iodine deficient. Brownstein says, "Iodine deficiency may be responsible for the epidemic increase in cancer of the breast (one in seven U.S. women currently have breast cancer), prostate, ovary, uterus, thyroid, and pancreas. Every one of the cancers listed is increasing at epidemic rates. There are a whole host of illnesses that are increasing at epidemic rates that may reflect falling iodine levels including ADHD, thyroid disorders including hypothyroidism and autoimmune thyroid problems, and cystic breasts."

In the analysis of National Health and Nutrition Examination Surveys, data of moderate to severe iodine deficiency is present now in a significant proportion of the U.S. population, with a clear increasing trend over the past 20 years, caused by reduced iodized table salt usage. Along with magnesium and selenium, iodine is one of the most deficient minerals in our bodies. Iodine is essential for the synthesis of thyroid hormone, but selenium-dependent enzymes (iodothyronine deiodinases) are also required for the conversion of thyroxine (T4) to the biologically active thyroid hormone, triiodothyronine (T3). Selenium is the primary mineral responsible for converting T4 to T3—essential thyroid hormones—in the liver.

Iodine is a vital micronutrient required at all stages of life with fetal life and early childhood being the most critical phases of requirement. Iodine is metabolized in the human body through a series of stages involving the hypothalamus, pituitary, thyroid gland, and blood.

Iodine can be used in many different ways depending on the clinical situation. It can be administered orally, applied transdermally (on the skin), vaporized in a nebulizer for application into the lungs, and used in douches.

Though officially recognized as the cure for goiter, the modern medical establishment has turned its back on using iodine to treat other diseases, even though iodine is the oldest allopathic medicine proven through 200 years of clinical use. Iodine does not cause problems in people, it cures disease through the fulfillment of nutritional law. Iodine is essential for human development and health. Iodine is detected in every organ and tissue in the body and is absolutely necessary for a healthy thyroid, as well as healthy ovaries, breasts, and prostate. Besides the increased risk for breast cancer in iodine deficient women, there is convincing evidence that iodine deficiency increases the risk of thyroid cancer.

Nothing replaces iodine. However, poisonous fluoride, bromide, and other halogen imitators step in as toxic substitutes, all of which mess up thyroid physiology. Moreover, nothing protects against radioactive isotopes of iodine more than natural iodine. The main causes of suppressed thyroid functions are *Candida*, mercury, fluoride, and a deficiency of iodine. Until 1970, doctors prescribed fluoride as thyroid-suppressing medication for patients with an over-active thyroid even though fluoride is a thyroid poison.

You cannot be a parent today and not have iodine in the house. All parents need to understand the importance of iodine and how to use it to protect their kids from the dangerous world of antibiotics and antibiotic resistant bacterial strains. Iodine gives parents protection against their doctors because of the diminished need for dangerous antibiotics and vaccines.

However, there is more to the story about why iodine has taken a backseat to drugs. The use of iodine goes back centuries, longer than anything else used by practitioners of modern medicine. Pharmaceutical medicine pushed its way into pharmacies and pushed out effective natural medicines like iodine and medical marijuana, two of the most popular medicines 100 years ago.

Medical textbooks contain several vital pieces of misinformation about the essential element iodine, which may have caused more human misery and death than both world wars combined.

—Dr. Guy E. Abraham, MD

According to Dr. Guy E. Abraham, founder of the Iodine Project, "The essential element iodine has been kept in the Dark Ages over the last 60 years after World War II. We need to remedy the gross neglect of this essential element by the medical profession, poorly represented in medical textbooks and vilified in endocrine publications." Dr. Abraham insisted rediscovering iodine as the universal medicine is crucial. Iodine held this esteemed position for over 100 years before World War II, and now we are finally coming to see we cannot live without it. Iodine is essential for survival in the 21st century.

Dr. Michael Zimmerman, in his article in *The Journal of Nutrition*, follows the history of iodine's use in modern science:

In 1811, Courtois noted a violet vapor arising from burning seaweed ash, and Gay-Lussac subsequently identified the vapor as iodine, a new element. The Swiss physician Coindet, in 1813, hypothesized the traditional treatment of goiter with seaweed was effective because of its iodine content and successfully treated goitrous patients with iodine. Two decades later, the French chemist Boussingault, working in the Andes Mountains, was the first to advocate prophylaxis with iodine-rich salt to prevent goiter. The French chemist Chatin was the first to publish, in 1851, the hypothesis that iodine deficiency was the cause of goiter. In 1883, Semon suggested myxedema was due to thyroid insufficiency and the link between goiter, myxedema, and iodine was established when, in 1896, Baumann and Roos discovered iodine in the thyroid. In the first 2 decades of the 20th century, pioneering studies by Swiss and American physicians demonstrated the efficacy of iodine prophylaxis in the prevention of goiter and cretinism. Switzerland's iodized salt program has been operating uninterrupted since 1922. Today, control of the iodine deficiency disorders is an integral part of most national nutrition strategies.

—Michael B. Zimmermann, Oxford Academic, Google Scholar

Some might say that the takeover by pharmaceutical medicine is a business driven science. Consider this: While the medical establishment treats patients with vaccines, psychiatric medicines, statin drugs, and antibiotics, these drugs have created a series of antibiotic resistant strains of bacteria that people are increasingly dying from. Hundreds of millions are slated to die from these infections over the next few decades, so it's better not to be caught flat-footed without iodine in the house.

Iodine is a protocol medicine, meaning it should be studied and used in the context of other similar basic medicines, that when combined with a number of other natural compounds give patients and doctors more medical power to fight disease. When we visit fine emergency rooms or intensive care wards, we discover the secrets they would hide from us. Secrets like magnesium chloride, sodium bicarbonate, and selenium, all used to save lives in a heartbeat. And in the same way, iodine is a bedrock medicine, meaning we cannot be healthy without it.

This book is designed to present a clear understanding of the healing properties of iodine. In Part 1 you will be introduced to the basics of iodine as a crucial medicine; its many roles in healing and preventing disease, and how iodine deficiency has been linked to major illnesses. It takes a look at iodine as a nutritional drug, a therapeutic agent, and the healing properties it contains. The section provides reasons to think of iodine as an anti-infectious super medicine, as a replacement for vaccines and antibiotics, and why it should be considered as a treatment for cancer.

Part 2 of the book sets the foundation for understanding and a guide for the proper use of iodine, and how iodine works to combat toxins (heavy metals and halogen poisons) in our body. It provides iodine product recommendations, iodine preparations, and applications, such as transdermal use, oral use, and iodine douches, as well as iodine dosages. This section also examines the dangers and risks of being exposed to radioactive iodine (I-129 and I-131) and the treatments and prevention of poisoning from radioactive iodine. You will see that iodine is one of the best antidotes for radiation poisoning.

In Part 3 you will take a closer look at certain conditions and related iodine treatments. It provides an understanding of the medicinal and biologic effects of iodine. It examines the causes of and iodine treatments and preventions for diseases related to the thyroid, cancers (breast cancer and skin cancer), and heart disease. You will also learn why pediatric iodine is a wiser choice that antibiotics and vaccines for childhood infections and viruses. This section also lays out the research that shows how iodine deficiency is related to fetal brain development and the importance of iodine sufficiency during pregnancy.

By the time you finish reading *Healing with Iodine,* you will be equipped with the knowledge of how and why iodine is a critical nutritional medicine and a nutrient the body needs in preventing and treating health problems. It is nutritional, but it is also one of the most effective medicines in the world. You will have a better understanding of why the medical community needs to focus on the importance of iodine sufficiency. The use of iodine provides the medical world with the most dramatic single thing you can do as a precaution and to restoring your well-being.

PART ONE
The Basics of Iodine

1. Iodine—
Crucial Medicine
for the 21st Century

This book is about iodine, one of the most useful medicinal substances that exist. Iodine is one of the only medicines that offers a clear cure for a specific disease—goiter. However, in this book you will find out that it is an essential medicine for the treatment of all diseases, including cancer. It will be a while still before one will commonly hear doctors recommending iodine and that is unfortunate. When it comes to cancer patients, they should be taking extremely high dosages.

Today many doctors are seeking alternatives and many alternative health care practitioners are in search of more powerful and safe ways of helping their patients. Iodine should satisfy everyone because it has the potential to help just about everyone who supplements with it. We all need iodine to survive, it is essential for human physiology so our health is dependent on its presence in sufficient quantities.

Iodine is not only necessary for the production of thyroid hormone;
it is also responsible for the production of all the other hormones in the body.

—Dr. David Brownstein, Medical Director, Bloomfield, Michigan

WHAT IS IODINE?

The molecular mass of iodine (126.90 U) is the highest of all the elements used in biological systems. This unique character is reflected in its atomic number: The proton count per atom for iodine (I 53) is significantly higher than any other common or essential trace element used by living organisms, including zinc (Zn 30) and iron (Fe 26).

Elemental iodine is easily reduced or oxidized. In its elemental state, iodine can be bound to carbon, oxygen, or hydrogen in organic molecules. The ease of these chemical reactions gives rise to a high diversity of ionic, iodine containing molecules. Ionic iodine can be found in different states of validity, often bound to oxygen or hydrogen. For instance, in the salt Potassium Iodide (KI), iodine is present with a negative validity (1–) in the ion I–. In the salt Potassium Iodiate (KIO3), iodine is molecularly bound to oxygen, and is present with a positive validity (5+) in the ion IO3. The reducing or oxidative properties of iodine containing molecules make them particularly suitable as catalysts in a wide range of chemical synthesis processes.

Governments around the world recognized iodine's importance many years ago and started putting it into salt. However, they forgot to tell everyone that iodine is volatile and evaporates fast. Therefore, we start with a minuscule amount in table salt and lose most of it as it sits on the table. The RDA and the amount of iodine put in salt is obscenely low—inadequate supply of our body's full need for iodine.

Though it was a good idea to put iodine in salt (in the old days iodine was added to bread instead of bromide), medical science and clinical experience indicate that we should be taking a lot more than the miserly amount we get from iodized salt. Low microgram dosages do not cover our needs for iodine, and the sooner doctors and patients wake up to this fact the better.

IMPORTANCE OF IODINE

Humans in the 21st century have an absolute need for iodine supplementation. Iodine is the only medicinal that stands between antibiotic resistance and us. There are many principal reasons we need iodine in abundance.

Iodine as an Anti-fungal and Antiviral

Iodine's antibiotic, anti-fungal, and antiviral effects go beyond antibiotics because it kills viruses, which antibiotics do not. Iodine kills fungus and yeast like *Candida*, which antibiotics do not. In addition, it does it without creating antibiotic resistant strains of bacteria. Scientists are also finding that antibiotics are causing bacteria to grow faster instead of killing them, so it is almost suicidal not to employ iodine as the first line of defense in our fight against infections.

The *Salon* magazine published, "Over 95 percent of physicians are concerned about antibiotic resistance," and that is all we need to know about iodine, which everyone should have on hand in their homes for everyday use as well as emergencies. Iodine has it all over antibiotics not only because it takes down viruses as well as fungus, but also because it does not provoke bacteria to become resistant to it.

Though it kills 90 percent of bacteria on the skin within 90 seconds, its use as an antibiotic has been tragically ignored. Iodine exhibits activity against bacteria, molds, yeasts, protozoa, and many viruses; indeed, of all antiseptic preparations suitable for direct use on humans and animals and upon tissues, only iodine is capable of killing all classes of pathogens. Most bacteria are killed within 15 to 30 seconds of contact.

Iodine, the antiseptic of all time.

—Dr. David Derry, author of *Breast Cancer & Iodine*

Iodine as a Treatment

The antiseptic properties of iodine are used to sterilize every surface and material in hospitals. Iodine is an excellent microbicide with a broad range of action. The minimum number of iodine molecules required to destroy one bacterium varies with the species. For H. influenzae it was calculated to be 15000 molecules of iodine per cell. When bacteria are treated with iodine, the inorganic phosphate up-take and oxygen consumption by the cells immediately ceases.

Dr. Derry says iodine is effective "for standard pathogens such as Staphylococcus, but also iodine has the broadest range of action, fewest side effects and no development of bacterial resistance." Some doctors have reported that it is excellent for the treatment of mononucleosis. Though iodine kills all single celled organisms it is not exploited for internal use by modern day physicians to combat internal infections.

Iodine is able to penetrate quickly through the cell walls of microorganisms.

Iodine was not available to simple life forms at the beginning of evolution; it was not until seaweed concentrated did it become involved in higher life forms. It is for this reason that the simplest level of life cannot tolerate iodine. Iodine kills by combining with the amino acids tyrosine or histidine. All single cells showing tyrosine on their outer cell membranes are killed instantly by a simple chemical reaction with iodine that denatures proteins.

Yeast Infections

Many women find after taking antibiotics they get vaginal yeast infections (because their normal bacterial balance has been lost). Antibiotics bring on fungal and yeast infections, thus will eventually be seen as one additional cause of cancer since more and more oncologists are seeing yeast and fungal infections as an integral part of cancer and its cause. With upwards of 40 percent of all cancers thought to be involved with and caused by infections, the subject of antibiotics and the need for something safer, more effective, and life serving is imperative.

A U.S. medical scientist says cancer—always believed to be caused by genetic cell mutations—can in reality be caused by infections from viruses, bacteria, yeasts, molds, and fungus parasites. "I believe that, conservatively, 15 to 20 percent of all cancer is caused by infections; however, the number could be larger—maybe double," said Dr. Andrew Dannenberg, director of the Cancer Center at New York-Presbyterian Hospital/Weill Cornell Medical Center. Dr. Dannenberg made the remarks in a speech in December 2007 at the annual international conference of the American Association for Cancer Research.

Iodine Prevents and Treats Cancer

Iodine is indispensable in protecting against thyroid cancer, breast cancer, ovarian cancer, as well as prostate cancer because all of these glands concentrate iodine more than other tissues. Deficiencies in iodine leave these glands vulnerable. Iodine also is indispensable for treating anything on the skin, even skin cancer, mainly because it kills everything on contact that does not belong. Studies have demonstrated a relationship between low iodine intake and fibrocystic disease of the breast (FDB), both in women and laboratory animals.

"Just how likely is an iodine deficiency in cancer? In an in-house study, 60 cancer patients (various types) were given the iodine-loading test and then measured for urinary excretion. All 60 patients were found to be seriously deficient in body stores of iodine and some had great excesses of bromine. The best case excreted only 50 percent of the load and the worst excreted only 20 percent (that means they were retaining a very high 80 percent). Folks, these are some serious numbers. One hundred percent of these cancer sufferers were deficient in iodine! I assure you the problem is population wide," writes Dr. Robert Rowen.

Breast tissue contains the body's third highest concentrations of this essential mineral, so shortfalls in iodine needs have a highly negative impact on breast tissue. Iodine shortfalls coupled with bromine and other toxic halogens cause fibrocystic breast disease and breast cancer.

High intake of iodine is associated with a lower risk of breast cancer. Low iodine intake is associated with liver cancer. Iodine is ideal for treating skin cancer. These are just the tip of the iceberg in terms of how important iodine is for cancer patients.

Iodine is recognized as an integral nutrient for proper immune function by the Institute of Medicine and as well as the United Nations Nutritional Policy Board. Dr. Rashid Buttar said, "Cancer first and foremost is a problem with the immune system. You cannot have cancer if you have an intact immune system." Some physicians believe that iodine is responsible for half of our immune system strength and response.

When we remember that infections cause many cancers and late stage infections go along with late stage cancer, and that iodine kills all kinds of pathogens on contact if enough is administrated, we come face to face with the fact that iodine is one of the most useful and essential substances for the prevention and treatment of cancer.

Iodine is important in cancer treatment, not only because it provokes cell apoptosis and kills viruses, bacteria, and fungus on contact, but also because *iodine is crucial in metabolism and oxygen deliver to the cells.* Any element that threatens the oxygen carrying capacity of the human body will promote cancer growth. Likewise, any therapy that improves the oxygen function can be expected to enhance the body's defenses against cancer. In order for cancer to 'establish' a foothold in the body, it has to be deprived of oxygen. If these two conditions can be reversed, cancer can not only be slowed down, but it can actually be cured. Iodine is a safe form of chemotherapy.

Iodine Is Protective Against Radioactive Iodine

Because iodine deficiency results in increased iodine trapping by the thyroid, iodine deficient individuals of all ages are more susceptible to radiation-induced thyroid cancer.

Iodine plays a crucial role in the body's elimination system by inducing apoptosis, or what is called programmed cell death. This is vital because this process is essential to growth and development and for destroying cells that represent a threat to the integrity of the organism, like cancer cells and cells infected with viruses.

Women with goiters (a visible, non-cancerous enlargement of the thyroid gland)
owing to iodine deficiency have been found to have a three times greater
incidence of breast cancer. A high intake of iodine is associated with a low
incidence breast cancer, and a low intake with a high incidence of breast cancer.

—Dr. Donald Miller Jr.

Dr. John W. Gofman, Professor Emeritus of Molecular and Cell Biology in the University of California at Berkeley, has written extensively about the effort to belittle the menace of low-level radiation. People associated with the nuclear and medical industries assert falsely, "There is no evidence that exposure to low-dose radiation causes any cancer—the risk is only *theoretical*," or "the risk is utterly *negligible*," or "the accidental exposures were below the *safe* level," and even "there is reasonably good evidence that exposure to low-dose radiation is *beneficial* and lowers the cancer rate." By any reasonable standard of scientific proof, the weight of the human evidence shows decisively that cancer is inducible by ionizing radiation even at the lowest *possible* dose and dose-rate—which means that the risk is never theoretical.

Different isotopes of radioactive iodine, one with an incredibly long half-life, have been dumped into the environment by the Fukushima meltdown. Iodine deficient adults and children are sitting ducks to their radioactive cousins especially if they are eating milk and cheese because radioactive iodine gets into the grass that the cattle eat and it just goes up the food chain to your door.

Iodine Metabolism

Iodine is also a necessity in metabolism. Human life is not possible without iodine. That truth is important to every cell in our bodies. It is of crucial importance for your health and well-being. The thyroid gland plays a main role in the metabolism of iodine. The metabolism of iodine occurs in three steps:

1. Iodine trapping is the first step. During this step iodide is transferred from the capillary into the follicular cell of the gland.

2. The second step is synthesis and secretion of the thyroglobulin. Thyroblobulin a large complex protein used to hold most of the iodine concentrated in the thyroid.

3. The oxidation of iodide is the third step. In this last step iodine atoms are

formed for the production of the thyroid hormones, thyroxine (T4), and triiodothyronine (T3).

Iodine's Role In The Production Of Hormones

Iodine is utilized by every hormone receptor in the body. The absence of iodine causes a hormonal dysfunction that can be seen with practically every hormone inside the body. Iodine helps synthesize thyroid hormones and prevents both hypo- and hyperthyroidism. Iodine sufficiency reverses hypo- and hyperthyroidism.

Iodine's ability to revive hormonal sensitivity seems to significantly improve insulin sensitivity. Iodine attaches to insulin receptors and improves glucose metabolism. Iodine is the best nutritional support for your thyroid. Your thyroid controls your metabolism and the efficiency of your metabolism is directly related to that of your immune system.

Iodine's Role in the Immune System

The body's ability to resist infection and disease is hindered by long-term deficiency in iodine. Poor immune response is directly tied in with impaired thyroid function; a deficiency in iodine can greatly affect the immune system because low levels of iodine lead to problems with the thyroid gland.

Iodine purifies water and it does the same job on the bloodstream. Iodine purifies the complete bloodstream of the body (something the thyroid does every 17 minutes) meaning sufficient levels of iodine, especially in children, keeps the body free of pathogens, no vaccines needed! Iodine's true role, as clearly making up as much as half of the body's immune system, has yet to be understood by doctors, but should be as the age of antibiotic resistant, fungal resistant, and viral medication resistant infections threaten the human race.

Iodide is accumulated during phagocytosis, the process of engulfing and ingesting bacteria and other foreign bodies. The iodide is attached to the bacteria and to proteins, creating iodoproteins, including monoiodotyrosine (T1). Sometimes, the thyroid hormones are utilized as the source of the iodide.

Dr. Gabriel Cousens, a holistic physician and expert on spiritual nutrition, lists many other important functions of iodine. Iodine offers dozens of under-utilized applications and should always be included when treating or preventing disease. Simply put, there are no bacteria, virus, or other microorganism that can survive or adapt to an iodine-rich environment.

- High doses of iodine may be used for wounds, bedsores, inflammatory and traumatic pain, and restoration of hair growth when applied topically.

- High doses of iodine may be used to reverse certain diseases.

- Iodine activates hormone receptors and helps prevent certain forms of cancer.

- Iodine decreases insulin needs in diabetics.

- Iodine deficiency is a global health threat.

- Iodine destroys pathogens, molds, fungi, parasites, and malaria.

- Iodine eliminates toxic halogens from the body (including radioactive I-131).

- Iodine helps in the diminishing of tissue scarring, cheloid formations, and Dupuytren's and Peyronie's contractures, which are hyper-scarring conditions.

- Iodine helps support protein synthesis.

- Iodine is anti-mucolytic (meaning it reduces mucus catarrh).

- Iodine is needed with the use of cordless phones, cell phones, and now smart meters to prevent hypothyroidism.

- Iodine makes us smarter.

- Iodine neutralizes hydroxyl ions and hydrates the cells.

- Iodine prevents fibrocystic breast disease.

- Iodine prevents heart disease.

- Iodine protects ATP function and enhances ATP production.

- Iodine regulates estrogen production in the ovaries.

- Iodine supports apoptosis.

- Iodine supports pregnancy (as the fetus undergoes more apoptosis than any other developmental stage).

- Iodine supports spiritual development.

CONCLUSION

Now that you have a better understanding of what iodine is and its benefits in fighting disease, let's turn our attention to the importance of iodine in producing thyroid hormone, in oxygen consumption, and in an oxygen-based metabolism.

2. *Iodine, Metabolism, and Oxygen*

Though doctors and people do not normally associate iodine with oxygen, in this chapter you will learn that iodine-carrying thyroid hormones are essential for oxygen-based metabolism. First, increases of iodine and thyroid hormones increase red blood cell mass and increase the oxygen disassociation from hemoglobin, the molecule in red blood cells that carries oxygen. Thyroid hormones have a significant influence on erythropoiesis, which is the process that produces red blood cells (erythrocytes).

THYROID DYSFUNCTIONS AND IODINE DEFICINCY

The most common thyroid dysfunctions, hypothyroidism and hyperthyroidism affect blood cells and cause anemia with different severity. Thyroid dysfunction and iodine deficiency induces other effects on blood cells, such as erythrocytosis (increase in number of red blood cells), leucopenia (decrease in number of white blood cells), thrombocytopenia (low blood platelet count), and in rare cases causes pancytopenia (a reduction in number of red and white blood cells and platelets). It also alters red blood cell (RBC) counts.

Thyroid hormone increase oxygen consumption, increase mitochondrial size, and the number and key mitochondrial enzymes. Meaning that iodine increases plasma membrane Na-K ATPase activity (the process of moving sodium and potassium ions across the cell membrance), increases futile thermogenic (fat burning) energy cycles, and decreases superoxide dismutase (enzyme found in almost all living cells) activity.

Thyroid hormones are known to play a major part in the regulation of mitochondrial oxidative metabolism.

Five Levels of Your Thyroid Hormone Pathway

Hypothyroidism and Hashimoto's thyroiditis are directly caused by a blockage at one or more levels of your thyroid hormone pathway.

Your thyroid gland:

- Thyroid peroxidase enzyme becomes inhibited, **blocking** your thyroid gland from producing thyroid hormone.

- Proteolyptic enzymes become suppressed, **blocking** your thryroid gland from secreting thyroid hormone.

Your liver:

- Diodenase enzyme becomes inhibited, **blocking** your liver from converting inactive T4 into active T3 causing you to become deficient in T3.

Your bloodstream:

- Thyroid transport proteins become **blocked** inside your bloodstream from carrying and delivering thyroid hormone to your cells.

Your cell receptors:

- Thyroid hormone cell receptors become **blocked**, preventing thyroid hormones from binding to and reaching your cells.

Your metabolism:

- Metabolism becomes **blocked**, preventing the mitochondria of your cells from metabolizing thyroid hormone and producing energy.

Mitochondria (cellular structures that power functions), by virtue of their biochemical functions, are a natural candidate as a direct target for the calorigenic effects (amount of heat generated) of thyroid hormones. Going further, we can see that mitochondria are highly dependent on thyroid hormones (thus iodine) for their very existence. Thyroid hormones are like the "signal" to make more mitochondria. Thyroid hormone (T3) has a profound effect on mitochondrial biogenesis; without T3, there will be less or no mitochondria. On the other hand, if mitochondria are damaged or depleted due to some reason other than too little T3, then existing T3 has "nothing to act on." You can have all the T3 in the world, but without mitochondria, there will not be any energy. Again, you can see the circular downward spiral of both host cell and mitochondria that can occur if either 1) too little or no T3 exists, or 2) too little or no mitochondria exist.

Summing it up we see that the total number of mitochondria in cells, and thus the total number of rechargeable ATP (Adenosine triphosphate) /ADP (Adenosine diphosphate) batteries, is dictated by the amount of functional thyroid hormone present in cells. If normal levels of thyroid hormone are reduced, the body develops hypothyroidism and the number of mitochondria in individual's cells is restricted.

Hypothyroidism is a very common condition that is implicated in what is called metabolic syndrome (formerly known as syndrome X). What is the basic cause of hypothyroidism? Iodine deficiency! Without iodine, the thyroid gland is unable to produce sufficient amounts of thyroid hormone. This leaves cells unable to function normally. In response, the body develops hypothyroidism.

OXYGEN-BASED METABOLISM
AND IODINE DEFICIENCY

Metabolism is defined as "taking food and converting it to energy." Our bodies need oxygen on a moment to moment basis and the higher the metabolism the more oxygen is needed. Cells will begin to rapidly deteriorate without adequate supply of oxygen or when the metabolism due to iodine deficiencies, go south. Efficiency of oxygen conversion into cellular energy is a key to the use of its energy; therefore, oxygen has in effect its own metabolism. The body's requirement for oxygen, makes oxygen the most important nutrient needed by the body.

Nutrients that are commonly used by animal and plant cells in respiration include sugar, amino acids, and fatty acids, and the most common oxidizing agent (electron acceptor) is molecular oxygen (O_2). Note that the amount of energy produced for the four types of food is roughly proportional to the amount of oxygen use, so that the metabolic rate can be measured by measuring the rate of oxygen consumption. Almost every process in the body that uses energy gets it from ATP, and in the process converts it to ADP.

The thyroid gland is like a building thermostat sending a message to a furnace to produce heat. Unlike a thermostat, the thyroid does not send its message to a single furnace, but, instead, sends the message to zillions of mitochondria via the chemical thyroxin that they should burn more fuel to create more biochemical energy. In order for the thyroid to send this "make more energy" message, the body needs ample amounts of iodine. There must be four atoms of iodine in each molecule of thyroxin (T4), the chemical that transmits the message to the mitochondria. Unfortunately, many people are deficient in iodine (because it is not in their food) with the result that the "make more energy" command is not communicated from the thyroid to the mitochondria. The consequence of this is low energy, low production of endorphins, and fat gain (because food energy is not converted to energy but is instead stored as fat).

Oxygen levels are sensitive to a myriad of influences. Toxicity, emotional stress, physical trauma, infections, reduction of atmospheric oxygen, nutritional status, lack of exercise, and especially improper breathing will affect the oxygen levels in our bodies. Now we have to see how important iodine and thyroid hormones are in this process as well.

IODINE, THYROID, OXYGEN, AND PH CONNECTION

Oxygen is our gasoline and our thyroid provides the spark. It is the spark plug that allows the flame of metabolism to be lit. Low thyroid increases oxygen cost, hinders metabolism, and forces us to breathe more, which increases the oxygen cost of breathing. We may get more energy immediately, which is good, but the oxygen cost is high. Our engine overworks to make up for the "dirty spark plugs" of our thyroid and parathyroid glands. A lack of thyroid hormones leads to a general decrease in the rate of utilization of fat, protein, and carbohydrate. The burning of our foods does not run cleanly when iodine is deficient.

Moreover, we find out that the rate of oxygen consumption of human leucocytes (cells in the blood that counteract foreign substances) is directly related to thyroid activity. Animal studies [Barker, 1955] show that the rate of oxygen uptake of many tissues is lowered by thyroidectomy and raised by administration of thyroid hormone. These tissues include liver, kidney, and skeletal and cardiac muscle.

Suiciding Healthy Oxygen Levels with Iodine Deficiency

When the oxygen levels in the cells drops below 60 percent, the respiration process of making energy changes into fermentation and presto we have a cancer cell. Normal cells can turn cancerous, not just because of DNA malformation but also because of oxygen deficiency. Dr. Ma Lan and Dr. Joel Wallach point out that one type of white blood cell kills cancer cells by injecting them with oxygen, creating hydrogen peroxide in the cells.

Thyroid hormones stimulate diverse metabolic activities in tissues, leading to an increase in basal metabolic rate. One consequence of this activity is to increase body heat production, which seems to result, at least in part, from increased oxygen consumption and rates of ATP hydrolysis. Since living organisms use molecular oxygen only for cellular respiration, the rate of oxygen consumption is directly related to the rate of ATP production. Common symptoms of hypothyroidism arising after early childhood include lethargy, fatigue, cold-intolerance, weakness, hair loss, and reproductive failure mirroring drops in ATP production and reduced oxygen utilization.

pH Balance and Iodine Utilization

The most important factor in creating proper pH is increasing oxygen because no wastes or toxins can leave the body without first combining with oxygen. The more alkaline you are, the more oxygen your fluids can hold and keep. Oxygen also buffers/oxidizes metabolic waste acids helping to keep you more alkaline. "The Secret of Life is both to feed and nourish the cells and let them flush their waste and toxins", according to Dr. Alexis Carrell, Nobel Prize recipient in 1912. Dr. Otto Warburg, also a Nobel Prize recipient, in 1931 and 1944, said, "If our internal environment was changed from an acidic oxygen deprived environment to an alkaline environment full of oxygen, viruses, bacteria, and fungus cannot live."

The position of the oxygen disassociation curve (ODC) is influenced directly by pH, core body temperature, and carbon dioxide pressure. According to Warburg, it is the increased amounts of carcinogens, toxicity, and pollution that cause cells to be unable to uptake oxygen efficiently. This is connected with over-acidity, which itself is created principally under low oxygen conditions.

Iodine, which is high up on the atomic scale, requires near perfect pH for its assimilation into the body. Iodine is crucial for proper functioning of the thyroid, but the thyroid does not get access to iodine unless the body pH is near perfect, as it usually is in the blood. Body mineral content and balances control the quantity of electricity in our bodies. The speed at which the electricity flows is controlled by the body's pH balance and in fact, pH and voltage are measurements of each other. When the pH balance goes off:

- *Enzymes* that are constructive can become destructive.

- *Microbes* in the blood can change shape, mutate, or become pathogenic.

- *Mineral* assimilation can get thrown off.

- *Organs* of the body can become compromised, like your brain or your heart.

- *Oxygen* delivery to the cells suffers.

There are complex biochemical processes taking place in the body constantly in an attempt to keep blood pH as near perfect as possible. These are known as the pH buffering systems. These buffering systems need a good balance of minerals to work effectively. If we are getting inadequate mineral intake from the food we eat, we are going to start having problems with our pH balancing systems.

Slightly alkaline intercellular fluids hold 10 to 20 times more oxygen than slightly acidic inter-cellular fluids. A pH 6.0 is ten times more acid than 7.0. pH; 5.0 is 100 times more acid; 4.0 is 1,000 times as acid; and so on. The body pH value tells you how acidic or alkaline your body is relative to a neutral 7.0, and balanced body pH is essential for a healthy body and a major line of defense against sickness and disease.

"Iodine's a great alkalinizing agent. It can elevate the pH. In those few patients I see with an alkalanized pH, iodine seams to lower the pH in them. Perhaps it's more of an adaptogen for pH than an alkalinizing agent," says Dr. David Brownstein, Medical Director of the Center for Holistic Medicine in West Bloomfield, Michigan. "We're seeing that iodine, so crucial to good health, may in fact be the ultimate adaptogen," says Nan Katherine Fuchs, PhD, in her book *The Health Detective's 456 Most Powerful Healing Secrets*. An adaptogen is a product that adapts to whatever is needed within the body. Specifically this means an adaptogen promotes homeostasis and stabilizes the processes of the body. It will normalize body functions.

The spread or metastases of cancer is inversely proportional to the amount of oxygen and the acidity around the cancer cells. The more oxygen, the slower the cancer spreads. The less oxygen and the higher the acidity the faster the cancer metastasizes. Oxygen is the enemy of cancer cells and so is iodine. Research scientists from the Cancer Research UK–MRC Gray Institute for Radiation Oncology and Biology at the University of Oxford have discovered that oxygen makes cancer cells weak and less resistant to treatment.

The most important factor in creating proper pH is increasing oxygen because no wastes or toxins can leave the body without first combining with oxygen. The more alkaline you are, the more oxygen your fluids can hold and keep. Oxygen also buffers/oxidizes metabolic waste acids helping to keep you more alkaline. Iodine sufficiency is one crucial key to oxygen sufficiency. According to Annelie Pompe, a prominent mountaineer and world-champion free diver, alkaline tissues can hold up to 20 times more oxygen than acidic ones. When our body cells and tissues are acidic (below pH of 6.5 to 7.0), they lose their ability to exchange oxygen. Increases of carbon dioxide, bicarbonates, and electrons lead to increased oxygen.

The quickest way to increase oxygen and pH is through the administration of sodium bicarbonate and that is why bicarbonate has always been a mainstay emergency room and intensive care medicine. Of course, when we increase oxygen and pH levels we are simultaneously increasing cellular voltage. We can violently pull the rug out from under most pathogens by bombarding them with a blast of alkalinity, which is the same thing as blasting with oxygen when we take high dosages of iodine, along with supplying our immune system with plenty of magnesium, selenium, and sulfur.

OXYGEN–A SOURCE OF GOOD HEALTH

Improving oxygen intake, uptake, and assimilation is critical to the body's energy and as an inhibitor to disease and decay. Movement and exercise invites a need for more oxygen. To digest and assimilate food uses up oxygen. Every bodily function uses up oxygen in varying degrees.

Dr. D. Treacher, physician at St. Thomas' Hospital in the U.K., and Dr. R. Leach, Professor of Science at Missouri University write, "Mammalian life and the bioenergetic processes that maintain cellular integrity depend on a continuous supply of oxygen to sustain aerobic metabolism. Reduced oxygen delivery and failure of cellular use of oxygen occur in various circumstances and if not recognized result in organ dysfunction and death. Prevention, early identification, and correction of tissue hypoxia are essential skills. An understanding of the key steps in oxygen transport within the body is essential to avoid tissue hypoxia. Although oxygen is the substrate that cells use in the greatest quantity and on which aerobic metabolism and cell integrity depend, the tissues have no storage system for oxygen. They rely on a continuous supply at a rate that precisely matches changing metabolic requirements. If this supply fails, even for a few minutes, tissue hypoxaemia may develop resulting in anaerobic metabolism and production of lactate."

Dr. Otto Warburg won the Nobel Prize in Medicine in 1931 for his discovery that cancer was anaerobic: cancer occurs in the absence of free oxygen. As innocuous as this discovery might seem, it is actually a startling and significant finding worthy of a Nobel Prize. What it means is that cancer is caused by a lack of free oxygen in the body and therefore, whatever causes this drop in free oxygen to occur is a root cause of cancers.

Hypoxemia or what might be called "blocked oxidation" is followed by fermentation of sugar in cells, which then leads to the primary condition upon which cancer, infectious, and inflammatory processes feed. Viruses are "anaerobic" creatures, which thrive in the absence of oxygen. Yeast, mold, and fungus live in an anaerobic environment. Most strains of harmful bacteria (and cancer cells) are anaerobic and are not comfortable in the presence of higher oxygen levels, so doctors will find cancer cells easier to kill when oxygen levels are increased.

IODINE AS AN ANTIOXIDANT

Research published in the scientific journal of the National Academy of Sciences in the U.S. reveal iodine's biological role as an inorganic antioxidant—the first to be described in a living system—pointing to the intriguing effects of iodine in scavenging free radicals in human blood cells. Scientists have determined that brown kelp, which boasts the highest concentration of iodide of any plant or animal, passively takes in this element from seawater, and then releases it when needed to detoxify harmful reactive oxygen species, which are generated by such external forces as pollution and intense light, as well as by internal metabolic processes.

Iodine plays an important role in fending off human health threats presented by free radicals. "It's the simplest antioxidant you could possibly find," Researcher Dr. George Luther notes. "When the kelp is exposed to stress, it dumps the iodide, which is easily converted into molecular iodine," he explains. "Molecular iodine goes into the atmosphere, where it helps form clouds that decrease the heat from the sun. It's one way of getting rid of ozone close to the ocean surface," Luther says. Large brown seaweeds, when under stress, release large quantities of inorganic iodine into the coastal atmosphere, where it can contribute to cloud formation, thus influencing climate.

Dr. Tina Kaczor, a neuropathic physician, writes, "Iodine has been proposed as a primitive antioxidant, with algae having an effective and perhaps necessary evolutionary role in squelching free radicals from the atmosphere. In humans, iodide has been shown to favorably affect serum antioxidant status. Iodide may be acting directly as an electron donor, squelching free radicals, such as hydroxyl radicals. It may also be acting indirectly through iodination of amino acids (for example, tyrosine and histidine) or fatty acids (arachadonic acid), rendering them less likely to be oxidized themselves.

Dr. Sebastiano Venturi, in *Evolution of Dietary Antioxidants: Role of Iodine*, makes it clear that iodine is a crucial antioxidant and apoptosis-inductor with anti-tumor and anti-atherosclerotic activity. When we supplement with iodine we will see increased antioxidant activity and immune system function.

The antioxidant biochemical mechanism of iodides is probably the most ancient mechanism of defense from poisonous reactive oxygen species.

—Dr. Sebastiano Venturi

Iodine Found in Kelp

Sea minerals in general are very helpful because the relative composition of the body is similar to the composition of the sea, where the first forms of life began. The sea is rich in iodine, about 60 micrograms per liter. Brown algae (seaweeds) accumulate iodine to more than 30,000 times the concentration of this element in seawater. Marine vegetation concentrates iodine for its antimicrobial and antioxidant properties.

Doctors involved with the Chernobyl nuclear plant catastrophe in 1989 used kelp for detoxification and thyroid gland rehabilitation, Modifilan (brown seaweed extract) helped thousands of nuclear plant workers and people in the area who were affected by the explosion because the iodine is protective against Strontium 90 and other toxicities.

The most important nutrient provided by kelp is iodine. Seaweed is noted for its ability to bind heavy metals and radioactive pollutants. Dr. Yukio Tanaka of the Gastrointestinal Research Lab at McGill University demonstrated that kelp may inhibit the absorption of lead, cadmium, and radioactive strontium (one of the most hazardous pollutants). Eighty to 90 percent of radioisotopes of Strontium 90 could be removed from the intestinal tract in the presence of seaweed. Iodine and the sodium alginates found in seaweed are the specific agents that do the chelation. So much Strontium 90 has been released by nuclear explosions, power plants, and nuclear weapons facilities that it is believed that every person has detectable levels in their bone tissue. Many cancers are attributable to this contamination.

"Seaweeds (iodine) have exceptional value in the treatment of *Candida* overgrowth. They contain selenium and other minerals necessary for rebuilding immunity; furthermore the rich iodine content is used by enzymes in the body to produce iodine-charged free radicals, which deactivate yeasts. Before the advent of anti-fungal drugs, iodine was the standard medical treatment for yeasts. When candidiasis is complicated with tumors or cancers, then seaweed is of additional benefit. Salt should normally be restricted during *Candida* overgrowth".

CONCLUSION

As you have learned in this chapter, iodine and oxygen are crucial to the healthy workings of the thyroid gland and the metabolic processes, as well as warding off viral and infectious disease. Also noted in this chapter is the crucial role iodine plays as an antioxidant. In the next chapter you will gain a better understanding of the role of iodine as an antioxidant.

3. *Iodine Deficiency*

Iodine deficiency was once considered a minor problem, causing goiter, an unsightly but seemingly benign cosmetic blemish. However, it is now known that the effects on the developing brain are much more deadly, and constitute a threat to the social and economic development of many countries. Low amounts of thyroid hormones in the blood due to lack of iodine to make them, give rise to high levels of the pituitary hormone TSH, which in turn stimulate abnormal growth of the thyroid gland, sometimes causing goiters.

Deficient iodine levels (low thyroid) can be at the base of many illness symptoms, or it can accompany and "hide" behind other degenerative diseases. The list of health complaints consistently associated with an under-functioning thyroid is long and shocking. Conditions include memory loss, depression, infertility, rheumatic pain, repeated infections, skin problems, migraines, anemia, constipation, and poor vision. The routine thyroid tests used today often do not detect low thyroid function.

Over 95 percent of my patients tested were deficient in iodine.

—Dr. David Brownstein

Dr. Guy Abraham, researcher and author of *The Iodine Project* articles, wrote, "One might go as far as imagining that there might even be a conspiracy to keep us iodine deficient, because if we are iodine deficient our will to resist is diminished, our apparent intellect, energy, and vitality are all diminished and we are significantly more vulnerable to thyroid malfunction, endocrine/hormonal imbalances, breast cancer, ovarian cancer

27

and prostate cancer. Many fine physicians are wondering why the RDA for iodine would be set so low, and why would many of the former sources of iodine be diminished or removed and replaced with things like bromides and fluorides that deplete iodine and offer no worthwhile compensation for the replacement?"

Medical iodophobia has reached pandemic proportions. It is highly contagious and has wreaked havoc on the practice of medicine and on the U.S. population.

—Dr. Guy Abraham

According to current W.H.O. (World Health Organization) statistics more than 3 billion people in the world live in iodine deficient countries and it is known that deficiencies of selenium, vitamin A, and iron may exacerbate the effects of iodine deficiency. In the analysis of "National Health and Nutrition Examination Surveys" data of moderate to severe iodine deficiency is present now in a significant proportion of the U.S. population, with a clear increasing trend over the past 20 years, caused by reduced iodized table salt usage.

IODINE IN FOOD

The most common statement you will find on many sites about iodine is, "Iodine deficiency is rare, because in most countries, iodine (as iodide) is added to commercial table salt." What they do not say is that the added iodine evaporates quickly from the salt leaving on trace amounts. In 1999, global health experts announced that iodine deficiency continues to be a serious threat to global health. Insufficient iodine is the most common—yet most preventable—cause of brain damage throughout the world, with 1.6 billion people at risk.

When the medical establishment calculates iodine deficiency, they are only looking at enough iodine to prevent goiter. Dr. Donald Miller, Jr., Professor Emeritus of Surgery at the University of Washington, reports, "People in the U.S. consume an average 240 micrograms (µg) of iodine a day. In contrast, people in Japan consume more than 12 milligrams (mg) of iodine a day (12,000 µg), a 50-fold greater amount. They eat seaweed, which include brown algae (kelp), red algae (nori sheets, with sushi), and green algae (chlorella). Compared to terrestrial plants, which contain only trace amounts of iodine (0.001 mg/gm), these marine plants have high concentrations of this nutrient (0.5 to 8.0 mg/gm). When studied in 1964,

Japanese seaweed consumption was found to be 4.5 grams (gm) a day and that eaten had a measured iodine concentration of 3.1 mg/gm of seaweed (= 13.8 mg of iodine). According to public health officials, mainland Japanese now consume 14.5 gm of seaweed a day (= 45 mg of iodine, if its iodine content, not measured, remains unchanged). Researchers have determined that residents on the coast of Hokkaido eat a quantity of seaweed sufficient to provide a daily iodine intake of 200 mg a day. Saltwater fish and shellfish contain iodine, but one would have to eat 15 to 25 pounds of fish to get 12 mg of iodine." Sources include most sea foods, (ocean fish, but not fresh fish, shellfish, especially oysters), unrefined sea salt, kelp and other sea weeds, fish broth, butter, pineapple, artichokes, asparagus, dark green vegetables, and eggs. Certain vegetables, such as cabbage and spinach, can block iodine absorption when eaten raw or unfermented and are called goitrogens. But eating fish won't give you iodine in mg amounts. To get 13.8 mg iodine, you would have to eat 10 to 20 pounds of fish per day.

Despite the widely held assumption that Americans are iodine-sufficient due to the availability of iodized salt, the U.S. population is actually at high risk for iodine insufficiency. Iodine intake has been decreasing in the U.S. since the early 70s as a result of changes in Americans' food and dietary habits, including the facts that iodized salt is infrequently used in restaurant and processed foods, and iodized salt sold for home use may provide far less than the amount of iodine listed on the container's label. The widespread dispersal of perchlorate, nitrate, and thiocyanate (competitive inhibitors of iodide uptake) in the environment

The Wolff-Chaikoff Effect

The Wolff–Chaikoff effect was discovered by Drs. Jan Wolff and Israel Lyon Chaikoff at the University of California. It is a temporary inhibition of thyroid hormone synthesis that supposedly occurs with increased iodine intake and is of no clinical significance, and an elevated TSH, when it occurs, is "subclinical." This means that no signs or symptoms of hypothyroidism accompany its rise. Some people taking milligram doses of iodine, usually more than 50 mg a day, develop mild swelling of the thyroid gland without symptoms. The vast majority of people, 98 to 99 percent, can take iodine in doses ranging from 10 to 200 mg a day without any clinically adverse affects on thyroid function.

blocks absorption of the little iodine Americans do consume, further compounding the problem.

Dr. Brice E. Vickery, a chiropractor, said, "I have seen that a couple of mgs of iodine daily will cure iodine deficiency in the person with adequate gut absorption powers. This will allow them to utilize their proteins; however it will not mean that they have full body iodine sufficiency (iodine receptors) in tissues, such as breast, uterus, prostate, skin, saliva glands, stomach, colon, choroid plexus, and eye. It will also not assure that a thyroid whose receptor space is taken up with another halogen, such as bromine or fluorine, will have a full sufficiency of iodine for hormone production."

SYMPTOMS

Iodine deficiency causes the same symptoms as an underactive thyroid gland, hypothyroidism (see page 18). In adults, such symptoms include:

- Brittle nails
- Cold hands and feet
- Constipation
- Depression
- Dry and scaly skin, puffy skin
- Edema
- Headaches

- Hoarse voice
- Impaired mental function
- Muscle cramps
- Myalgia
- Poor memory
- Sparse and coarse hair
- Weakness
- Weight gain

RISKS

Doctors agree that a lack of iodine in the diet causes a spectrum of disorders that includes, in increasing order of severity, goiter and hypothyroidism, mental retardation, and cretinism (severe mental retardation accompanied by physical deformities). Iodine deficient humans, like endemic cretins, suffer physical, neurological, mental, immune, and reproductive diseases. Iodine is important in the proper function of the nervous system and Dr. S. Cunnane, a cardiologist, suggests that "iodine is the primary brain selective nutrient in human brain evolution."

Cretinism

Cretinism is a condition associated with iodine deficiency and goitre, commonly characterized by mental deficiency, deaf-mutism, squint, disorders of stance and gait, stunted growth and hypothyroidism. In *Pediatrics:* American Academy of Pediatrics (1974), Paracelsus was the first to point out the relation between goitrous parents and mentally retarded children. As a result of restricted diet, isolation, intermarriage, as well as low iodine content in their food, children often had peculiar stunted bodies and retarded mental faculties, a condition later known to be associated with thyroid deficiency. Diderot in his 1754 Encyclopédie described these patients as "crétins". In French, the term "crétin des Alpes" also became current, since the condition was observed in remote valleys of the Alps in particular. The word cretin appeared in English in 1779.

Goiters

When iodine is deficient, the thyroid gland enlarges, forming a goiter, as it attempts to capture more iodine for the production of thyroid hormones. A goiter results from a lack of iodine in the diet. If the goiter arises from a deficiency of iodine in the food or water of a particular area, it's called an endemic goiter. Associated signs and symptoms of an endemic goiter include dysphagia, dyspnea, and tracheal deviation.

For Children

Iodine deficiency is a major cause of under-functioning intellect. Dr. Flechas, a family medicine practioner, agrees, "In newborn children iodine is responsible for the development of the babies' I.Q. Recent research shows iodine deficiency is felt to be the source of attention deficit disorder in children." We have an absolute epidemic of autism in this country," said Representative Dan Burton (R-Indiana). "Parents and doctors are struggling to find appropriate treatment options." What help iodine can be to neurological damaged children has not been explored yet, but iodine and magnesium logically should be some of the first things parents should reach for. We certainly will find science to create a foundation for the use of iodine before, during, and after pregnancy.

Children with iodine deficiency and its resulting hypothyroidism suffer from stunted growth, with mental retardation, and problems in movement, speech or hearing. Iodine deficiency is the single most common cause of preventable mental retardation and brain damage in the world. Iodine deficiency also decreases child survival. Children with IDD can grow up stunted, apathetic, mentally retarded, and incapable of normal movements, speech or hearing. If a nuclear radiation accident occurs, iodine deficiency increases the risk of thyroid cancer in children because the deficient thyroid gland collects the radioactive iodine.

For Pregnant Women

If a pregnant woman has this deficiency, the growth and brain development of the fetus may be abnormal. Unless the baby is treated soon after birth, mental retardation with short stature (cretinism) develops. Iodine deficiency in pregnant women causes miscarriages, stillbirths, and other complications.

Deficiency of iodine seems to cause more damage in developing embryos and in fact, in pregnant women iodine deficiency causes abortions and stillborns. It is not cretinism alone that holds risks from deficiency but the very survival of the infant itself. Adequate iodine may also provide protection from infection and vaccine damage. In a study done on 617 infants between the ages of 6 weeks and 6 months, in an iodine deficient area, it was shown that with the addition of 100 mg of iodine oil to the diet of newborns, that the death rate of infants was markedly lower than for those without any supplementation.

Mental Retardation

Iodine deficiency is the leading cause of mental retardation, producing typical reductions in IQ of 10 to 15 points. It has been speculated that deficiency of iodine and other micronutrients may be a possible factor in observed differences in IQ between ethnic groups.

Reproductive Risks

Iodine deficiency poses significant additional reproductive risks, including overt hypothyroidism and infertility. Hypothyroidism causes anovulation, infertility, and gestational hypertension. Adequate tissue iodine helps guide estrogen into friendly pathways that support proper function of female sex hormones. Iodine contributes to the formation of testosterone. In women this supports healthy sex drive. In men, testosterone is vital to function.

IODINE TESTING

A Swiss physician, Jean Surbeck, reports in the Price-Pottinger Nutrition Foundation newsletter that there is a simple home test to check your body's iodine level. He suggests taking a Q-Tip and painting an area about the size of a silver dollar with 2 percent tincture of iodine (from the drug store–get the kind that is not discolored). Since iodine will stain the skin yellow, you might want to paint it on your thigh.

If your iodine level is below normal, any iodine painted on the skin will disappear relatively quickly. By morning no evidence of it will remain. In practice the quicker the iodine disappears the more desperate the body is for iodine. Such a test varies considerably depending on the type of iodine used, where, and how much it is used.

My experience is that the atomic (nascent) iodine drops quickly through the skin when a person is deficient, which is another indication of its special properties. If the iodine just sits on the skin and stays wet you know the body is not needing or wanting any more iodine. This I have never seen happen!

CONCLUSION

Running our bodies without sufficient minerals is like running a car without oil. Our engines of cellular life begin to seize up today because of all the impurities in our food, air, water, and medical and dental drugs and substances. This chapter addressed the importance of iodine in your diet and the risks taken when you are iodine deficient. Read on to discover how iodine is an anti-infectious supplement.

4. *Iodine Is an Anti-Infectious Super Medicine*

In a world showing increases in infectious disease, antibiotic resistant bacteria, life-threatening inflammatory reactions triggered by fungal infections and dangerous antiviral drugs, and vaccines, we find iodine as the single most important mineral medicine that every man, woman, and child should be supplementing with at reasonably high dosages. Iodine happens to be mission critical for strong immune system response.

The Review on Antimicrobial Resistance (AMR) determined that, left unchecked, in the next 35 years, antimicrobial resistance could kill 300,000,000 people worldwide and stunt global economic output by $100 trillion. There are no other diseases we currently know of except pandemic influenza that could make that claim. In fact, if the current trend is not altered, antimicrobial resistance could become the world's single greatest killer, surpassing heart disease or cancer.

Four years ago the *Guardian* in England wrote, "Are you ready for a world without antibiotics. Antibiotics are the bedrock of modern medicine. But in the very near future, we're going to have to learn to live without them once again. And it's going to get nasty. The era of antibiotics is coming to a close. In just a couple of generations, what once appeared to be miracle medicines have been beaten into ineffectiveness by the bacteria they were designed to knock out. Once, scientists hailed the end of infectious diseases. Now, the post-antibiotic apocalypse is within sight."

More than 95 percent of the 500 physicians surveyed in a new Consumer Reports National Research Center poll are concerned about the growing problem of antibiotic-resistant infections. Over the previous 12 months, 85 percent of them treated a patient with a suspected or confirmed case of such an infection; 35 percent of those said their patient suffered significant complications or died as a result.

Called a global threat by the World Health Organization and "the next pandemic" by CDC (Center of Disease) director Thomas Friedan, antibiotic resistance threatens their ability to do their jobs. Imagine being a doctor and having to tell a patient with a common but serious disease, like pneumonia, a urinary tract infection, or gonorrhea, that there's nothing you can do to help them." Except that would be a ridiculous thing to say, because with iodine there is a lot a doctor or mother can do to help patients and loved ones.

WHY WE NEED IODINE NOW

The *New York Times* has a distressing report on the epidemic of antibiotic resistant "superbugs" killing newborns by the tens of thousands in India. "A deadly epidemic that could have global implications is quietly sweeping India, and among its many victims are tens of thousands of newborns dying because once-miraculous cures no longer work. These infants are born with bacterial infections that are resistant to most known antibiotics, and more than 58,000 died last year as a result, a recent study found.

"Five years ago, we almost never saw these kinds of infections," said Dr. Neelam Kler, chairperson of the department of neonatology at New Delhi's Sir Ganga Ram Hospital, one of India's most prestigious private hospitals. "Now, close to 100 percent of the babies referred to us have multidrug resistant infections. It's scary."

We do not have to look far to see why this is happening in India and destined to continue to spread around the world. Massive amounts of pharmaceutical waste—up to thousands of tons a day—are entering waterways near bulk drug manufacturing facilities in India. Researchers tested nearly 30 water samples near such facilities and all were contaminated with antimicrobials at levels up to 5,500 times higher than the environmental regulation limit. More than 95 percent of the samples also contained multidrug-resistant bacteria and fungi.

Antiviral Drugs and Antibiotics Damage Body Cells

Influenza's ability to resist the effects of popular antiviral agents should serve as a cautionary tale about U.S. plans to use the antiviral medications in the event of widespread avian flu infection. Researchers already know that widespread antiviral drug use can accelerate the evolution of drug resistance in viruses, and that resistant strains can emerge and spread rapidly. Iodine is needed in the world today more than it has ever been needed. Iodine is necessary when dealing with deadly viruses and would go a long way in decreasing the death rate from all of them; no pharmaceutical company or vaccine needed.

Side effects have been associated with the use of flu antiviral drugs, including nausea, vomiting, dizziness, runny or stuffy nose, cough, diarrhea, headache, and some behavioral side effects. These are the main symptoms of a bad cold or flu so it is not too far-fetched that the medications cause what they are supposed to prevent just as standard cancer treatments cause cancer.

Studies have shown that the chances of dying from hospital pneumonia or septicemia (blood poisoning) are twice as high if the bacteria are drug-resistant, rising in the case of pneumonia from 20 to 30 percent to 40 to 60 percent.

Many people who die in the hospital after surgery are dying not from the surgery itself but from the infections that have gotten out of control. "In many ways, this is it," Professor Tim Walsh. "This is potentially the end. There are no antibiotics in the pipeline that have activity against NDM 1-producing enterobacteriaceae. We have a bleak window of maybe 10 years where we are going to have to use the antibiotics we have very wisely, but also grapple with the reality that we have nothing to treat these infections with." Walsh, like most doctors today, has totally forgotten about iodine and how it is used routinely to sweep anything it is applied to clean of infections.

Highly contagious, spread by coughs and sneezes, pertussis is now epidemic in California, with 2,774 confirmed cases in 2010—a sevenfold increase from last year, putting the state on track for the worst outbreak in 50 years. Seven infants have died. Mothers everywhere are going to be desperate as this spreads further year by year. They are going to need to understand how to use iodine as well as magnesium and sodium bicarbonate to combat these vaccine failed infections. We have to hope that pediatricians will come to their senses and embrace safe ways of dealing with their patients' infections.

It may be some time before we really enter the predicted "post antibiotic era" in which common infections are frequently untreatable.
—Dr. Marc Lipsitch et al. Harvard School of Public Health

Iodine Is a Viral, Bacterial, and Fungal Killer

In the beginning of 2017, nearly three dozen people in the United States have been diagnosed with a deadly and highly drug-resistant fungal infection that has been rapidly spreading around the world. The fungus is a strain of a kind of yeast known as *Candida auris*. Unlike garden-variety yeast infections, this one causes serious bloodstream infections, spreads easily from person to person in health-care settings, and survives for months on skin and for weeks on bed rails, chairs, and other hospital equipment. Some strains are resistant to all three major classes of antifungal drugs. Up to 60 percent of people with these infections have died. The fact that *Candida auris* has an uncanny and dangerous ability to exploit cells around it is one of the main reasons we should return to iodine as our favored broad-spectrum antibiotic, antiviral, and anti-fungal agent. Iodine provides us with a safe way to strengthen innate responses to invading microbes while simultaneously correcting or eliminating a basic nutritional deficiency that causes immunological unresponsiveness. Iodine also chelates out mercury of the thyroid as well as the full list of halogens that are poisoning most everyone.

Dr. David Derry wrote, "Iodine was the most effective agent for killing viruses, especially influenza viruses. Aerosol iodine was found to kill viruses in sprayed mists, and solutions of iodine were equally effective. In 1945, Burnet and Stone found that putting iodine on mice snouts prevented the mice from being infected with live influenza virus in mists. They suggested that impregnating masks with iodine would help stop viral spread. They also recommended that medical personnel have iodine-aerosol-treated rooms for examination and treatment of highly infected patients. Current methods of dealing with influenza infection are isolation, hand washing, antiviral drugs, and vaccinations. All of these methods can be improved by incorporating iodine into them. When impregnated with iodine, masks become much more effective, and hand washing is more effect when done with mild iodine solutions."

Viral infections always have doctors scrambling because they have forgotten how effective iodine is against them. Dr. Richard Kunin, after 50 years of practice concluded that iodide destroys the virus of herpes. Both oral and genital lesions are treatable this way.

Research at the Massachusetts General Hospital tells us, "HIV was completely inactivated and could no longer replicate after exposure to the povidone-iodine preparations even at very low concentrations." Dr. Eliot Dick observed a 50 percent reduction in respiratory illnesses when using iodine. Many reports by patients find that a gargle of ten drops of potassium iodide in a glass of water, with or without additional vitamin C, relieved sore throat in a matter of hours.

The *Science Daily* reports, "With infectious diseases, it is often not the pathogen itself, but rather an excessive inflammatory immune response (sepsis) that contributes to the patient's death, for instance as a result of organ damage. On intensive care units, sepsis is the second-most common cause of death worldwide. In patients with a severely compromised immune system specially, life-threatening *Candida* fungal infections represent a high risk of sepsis." *Science Daily* informs us that, "Infectious diseases are the world's number-one cause of death, with pathogenic fungi being responsible for extremely dangerous infections. Worldwide, more than 6 billion are spent each year on anti-fungal medications, and the total costs of the medical treatment of infectious diseases caused by pathogenic fungi are estimated in the order of hundreds of billions of Euros." This is all highly unnecessary because sodium bicarbonate (baking soda) happens to be the best anti-fungal there is. Iodine, its cofactor selenium, and sodium bicarbonate are a killer combination against viruses, bacteria, and fungal infections.

IODINE REPLACES VACCINES AND ANTIBIOTICS

Pharmaceutical medicine is becoming impotent in the age of antibiotic resistant infections. It always has had difficulty treating fungal infections and vaccines are not halting the rise in viral infections that often, if you believe the CDC, lead to death. Iodine is the super hero medicinal able to take on infections of all types. All one has to do is reach for a bottle of iodine and mix it with water. First sign of sore throat or fever run for the iodine and gargle with iodine.

Dr. David Brownstein says that iodine is number one in his protocol. When one considers how important iodine is in preventing cancer, we would, if we were thinking straight, take daily iodine supplementation seriously. When a parent considers that iodine ensures, from the first sign of any problem with their kids, security because iodine is standing inches away, ready to take out infectious marauders on contact, they would consider iodine medicine more earnestly.

When we see that infections themselves frequently lead to cancer, then we do have to stop and consider why we are not taking iodine. Are you ready for a world without antibiotics? I am because my house always has a big stock of iodine. With iodine, there is a lot a doctor or mother can do to help people resist infections and cancer. Iodine/iodide is the super medicine we need in the 21st century if we do not want to be slaughtered as public health officials and medical scientists are promising. Iodine is just waiting, is already on the shelves and easily obtained on the Internet and comes in many forms for many uses.

Iodine is available in every pharmacy in the world. However, the common inexpensive form found there cannot be taken orally though it can be used for skin infections and skin cancer as well as systemic supplementation by getting in moderate dosages through the skin.

Medications May Cause Adverse Effects

Many physicians are unaware of lasting adverse effects caused by routinely prescribed medications, such as antibiotics. Antibiotic therapy for minor colds and runny noses is a common practice. People routinely receive multiple courses of broad-spectrum antibiotics throughout life or are injected with long-acting corticosteroid medicine for joint or muscle pain. Once established, sub-clinical colonization with yeast in the body may persist unrecognized for many years.

Antibiotics, such as tetracycline, can greatly increase yeast in the colon after only a few days. The extensive use of antibiotics will make the condition of *Candida* much worse because it reduces heavy metal excretion.

In 2005 a study the antibiotic Augmentin TM has been implicated in the formation of autism. The study strongly suggests the possibility of ammonia poisoning as a result of young children taking Augmentin. Augmentin has been given to children since the late 1980's for bacterial infections.

Antibiotics may be to blame for hundreds of children developing autism after having the controversial MMR jab. More than two-thirds of youngsters with the condition received four or more antibiotics in their first year, a British survey has revealed. It is thought the drugs weakened their immune systems, leaving them unable to withstand the impact of the triple jab.

Many physicians seem to be unaware that birth control pills comprised of the hormones estrogen and progesterone can also make the body more susceptible to fungal infections. If antibiotics are prescribed it acts as a double whammy to ensuring a fungal infection will take hold by diminishing the protective bacteria in the intestines.

Many pregnant women seek medical treatment for minor problems and are indiscriminately given antibiotics. This begins a long decline into problems that are complicated at each turn by OBGYN doctors at birth and by pediatricians who just love to poison children with the toxic chemicals found in vaccines. In many places in the world they still give mercury containing Hep B shots at birth.

Antibiotics are mostly derived from fungi and are therefore classified as mycotoxins. Mycotoxins are poisons.

Wrong Notions of Antibiotics

It is interesting to note that a new study is saying that the rule that patients must finish an antibiotics course is wrong. Telling patients to stop taking antibiotics when they feel better may be preferable to instructing them to finish the course, according to a group of experts who argue that the rule long embedded in the minds of doctors and the public is wrong and should be overturned. Consumption of antibiotics rose 36 percent between 2000 and 2010.

Some are urging the British government to wake up to the fact that, without effective antibiotics, we could see an end to life-saving transplants, chemotherapy, and routine operations, such as caesareans and hip replacements; and that continued misuse and overuse of antibiotics could, within a generation, see the global death toll from drug-resistant infections rise—more than currently die of cancer.

If we fail to act, we are looking at an almost unthinkable scenario where antibiotics no longer work and we are cast back into the dark ages of medicine where treatable infections and injuries will kill once again (David Cameron, Prime Minister). The reasons to get serious about iodine never end. Antibiotics add, on average, twenty years to our lives and so will iodine. For over seventy years, since the manufacture of penicillin in 1943, we have survived extraordinary operations and life-threatening infections. We are so familiar with these wonder drugs that we take them for granted. The truth is that we have been abusing them: as patients, as doctors, in our food.

More Reasons to Think Iodine Over Antibiotics

According to several studies, obstetricians and gynecologists write 2,645,000 antibiotic prescriptions every week. Internists prescribe 1,416,000 per week. This works out to 211,172,000 prescriptions annually in the United States, just for these two specialties. Pediatricians prescribe over $500 million worth of antibiotics annually just for one condition, ear infections. Yet topical povidone iodine (PVP-I) is as effective as topical ciprofloxacin, with a superior advantage of having no in vitro drug resistance and the added benefit of reduced cost of treatment.

Eventually antibiotics are going to be seen as one of the worst things to ever come out of pharmaceutical science because in the end they have made us only weaker in the face of ever increasingly strong super bugs that are resistant to all the antibiotics doctors have at their disposal. When we look at how deep the rabbit hole goes with antibiotics it will sicken our souls. Antibiotics have fulfilled their anti–biotic anti-life role leaving a long trail of death and suffering in the wake of their use.

Dr. Lisa Landymore-Lim wrote all about this in her book *Poisonous Prescriptions* asking, 'Do Antibiotics Cause Asthma and Diabetes?' We are now even beginning to question the role of antibiotics as a cause of cancer since they do lead to pathogen overgrowth especially in the area of yeast and fungi. Chris Woollams writes, "It is estimated that 70 per cent of the British population have a yeast infection. The primary cause of this is our love of antibiotics. Swollen glands? Take antibiotics. Tonsillitis? Take antibiotics."

Two studies in the recent past have shown an association between the uses of antibiotics with higher incidence of breast cancer. In one study, the increased risk was small, and the importance of the link has been played down by UK breast-cancer experts, but the findings add weight to recent studies that have found links between antibiotics and other diseases. In the past few years heavy antibiotic use has been linked to the inflammatory bowel disorder, Crohn's disease, and to children developing allergies, such as hayfever and asthma. And as we shall see antibiotics play a hidden role in autism and other neurological diseases.

The *Journal of the American Medical Association* has reported a study on 10,000 women in which women who took over 500 days of antibiotics in a 17 year period (dubbed 25 plus doses) had twice the risk of breast cancer as those that took none at all. Even women taking just one had a statistical risk increase to 1.5 times.1[vii] One reason we are losing the war on cancer is that antibiotics are doing their job too well and we are using them way too much. When we look at the available options to their use we discover that it is best to avoid their use except in extreme medical circumstances.

"We know that antimicrobial resistance will follow antimicrobial use as sure as night follows day," said Dr. John A. Jernigan, deputy chief of prevention and response from the Center of Disease Control. "It's just a biological phenomenon." It turns out that the indiscriminate killing of harmless microbes damages the body in complex ways we are only beginning to understand. Powerful antibiotics introduced into the complex environment in our intestines cause mayhem, much like a series of bombs tossed into a market square. Antibiotic resistance is a widespread problem, and one that the U.S. Centers for Disease Control and Prevention calls "one of the world's most pressing public health problems."

Resistant Bacteria In Chickens

A 17-year-old St Margaret's College student in New Zealand has exposed multiple antibiotic-resistant bugs in fresh chicken sold in supermarkets. Jane Millar's discovery of a range of resistant bacteria in chickens is an important finding that the bacteria have developed resistance to antibiotics not used in the poultry industry but important for treating serious infections in humans.

Jane bought six fresh chickens—free-range, barn-raised, and organic—from a supermarket. She took samples from each bird and grew bug colonies, which she used to test different antibiotics. Apramycin is an antibiotic used sparingly by the New Zealand poultry industry to treat infections. The bacteria of two chickens tested resistant to Apramycin. They also proved resistant to another two antibiotics from the same family—gentamicin and tobramycin—used for serious human infections. Gentamicin is not used by the poultry industry; tobramycin is restricted to human use only.

A recent risk assessment study commissioned by the U.S. Food and Drug Administration (FDA) has estimated that about 8,000 to 10,000 persons in the U.S. each year acquire fluoroquinolone-resistant *Campylobacter* infections from chicken and attempt to treat those infections with a fluoroquinolone.

One of the deadliest germs is a staph bacteria called M.R.S.A., short for methicillin-resistant *Staphylococcus aureus,* which lives harmlessly on the skin but causes havoc when it enters the body. Patients who do survive M.R.S.A. often spend months in the hospital and endure several operations to cut out infected tissue. Hospitalizations associated with a drug-resistant form of a *Staphylococcus* bacterium doubled over six years in the U.S. to nearly 280,000 cases in 2005. The death toll rose from 4,700 in 1999 to about 6,600 in 2005. It estimated that 94,000 Americans suffered invasive MRSA infections in 2005 and that about 19,000 died. "Recently there has been an alarming epidemic caused by community-associated (CA)-MRSA strains, which can cause severe infections that can result in necrotizing fasciitis or even death in otherwise healthy adults outside of healthcare settings," is the word coming from the National Institute of Allergy and Infectious Diseases (NIAID) research team, headed by Dr. Michael Otto. Necrotizing fasciitis is the so-called flesh-eating disease that can destroy healthy tissue.

Every day, new strains of bacteria, fungi, and other pathogenic
microorganisms are becoming resistant to the antibiotics
that once dispatched them with extreme prejudice.

One out of every 20 patients contracts an infection during a hospital stay in the U.S. Hospital infections kill an estimated 103,000 people in the United States a year, as many as AIDS, breast cancer and auto accidents combined. The vast majority of lethal cases occur in hospitals and nursing homes, where open wounds and punctures provide the opportunistic staph a ready path to the bloodstream and organs. The dangers of infection are worsening as many hospital infections can no longer be cured with common antibiotics.

VIRAL HYSTERIA

Doctors tend to get hysterical about viruses and antibiotic resistant bacteria because they refused to learn about and use the best and safest treatments for them, which is iodine. As early as June 1, 1905 an article was printed in the *New York Times* about the successful use of iodine for consumption/tuberculosis.

As public health officials struggle to track and contain a respiratory virus that has
hospitalized hundreds of children across the U.S., there are now concerns that
enterovirus D68 may also cause paralysis in some cases and death in others.

Samples collected from four patients who recently died have tested positive for enterovirus D68, according to the Centers for Disease Control and Prevention. These patients are not being given iodine.

The enterovirus is related to the common cold, and this strain has hit children hardest. Most only experience symptoms, such as a runny nose, though a small percentage develop trouble breathing and have to be admitted to the intensive care unit. The possibility of paralysis adds another layer to the mystery around the virus as it has spread across the nation and why it has caused such severe illness in so many children. Why are they not given iodine?

There have been 500 cases of children infected with this virus throughout 42 states thus far. At Children's Hospital Colorado, Dr. Chris Nyquist, the hospital's director of infection prevention and control said, "The current virus that is circulating has no antiviral medicine or vaccine so the common sense things are very important." What is more common sense then administering high dosages of magnesium chloride, sodium bicarbonate, and iodine to fight infections?

Viral Doubters

In this section we will see that the Measles virus has never been proven to exist and many doubt the existence of the HIV virus. Dr. Stefan Lanka, virologist and molecular biologist said, "So for a long time I studied virology, from the end to the beginning, from the beginning to the end, to be absolutely sure that there was no such thing as HIV. And it was easy for me to be sure about this because I realized that the whole group of viruses to which HIV is said to belong, the retroviruses—as well as other viruses which are claimed to be very dangerous—in fact do not exist at all."

Dr. Lanka reminds us, "Those side effects which are noted on the instruction slips accompanying packages of Tamiflu are almost identical to the symptoms of serious influenza. Thus, on a large scale, medicines are now being stored which cause precisely the same symptoms as those which appear in an actual so-called influenza. If Tamiflu is administered to sick persons, then this is likely to cause far more serious symptoms than those of a serious influenza. If a pandemic is stated to exist, then many people will take this medicine at the same time. In that case we will actually have unequivocal symptoms of a Tamiflu epidemic. Then deaths caused by Tamiflu are to be expected, and this will then be presented as evidence of the dangerous nature of the bird (or now swine) flu."

"We live with an uncountable number of retroviruses. They're everywhere—and they probably have been here as long as the human race," says Dr. Kary Mullis. Dr. Lanka adds, "It is being maintained that these short pieces of genetic material, which in the sense of genetics are not complete and which do not even suffice for defining a gene, together would make up the entire gene substance of an influenza virus."

BIOFILMS

Dr. Paul Yanick, Jr., a board-certified naturopath, has published in the Townsend Letter a very interesting work on infectious biofilms. Bacterial biofilms are ubiquitous in human physiology. They can crop up anywhere; we could call them bacterial slime for that is exactly what they are. Biofilms confront us daily in our mouths with the formation of dental plaque. It's very similar to the type of slime that grows inside a flower vase after two or three days.

> *Biofilms are in all chronic infections.*
> —Dr. J.W. Costerton, Montana State University

Dr. Yanick says, "There are certain kinds of pathogens that enter the cells via abnormalities of key cell membrane receptors—settling down into anaerobic tissue sites as a mucous-like and sticky matrix where it aggregates, communicates, and constructs slimy edifices called biofilms. Biofilms consist of a dense symbiotic aggregation of microbes embedded in a highly hydrated polymer, polysaccharide matrix of its own secretion, they often end up in the cornea, tonsils, wounds, nasopharynx, middle ear, prostate and urinary tract, teeth (under root canals, fillings, implants, or as chronic bacterial ostitis in extraction sites), dental plaque, oral soft tissues, gall bladder, GI epithelium, heart (endocarditis) and lungs, making them notoriously difficult to treat. Their anti-microbial resistance coupled with the inaccuracy of current lab tests to diagnose hidden biofilms and intracellular infections makes biofilms one of the greatest clinical challenges facing doctors today."

The mutational and transformational realities of pathogens provide reason to conclude iodine as the strong man to turn to in the antiviral, antibacterial, and antifungal pharmacy. Biofilm-related infections are involved in the deterioration of gums, ear infections, stubborn sinus infections, and chronic gall bladder and cardiac infections, just to mention a few of the possibilities. Iodine naturally is a solution, as is sodium bicarbonate, for breaking up biofilms.

Even in the healthy immune system, the unleashing of its magnificent and diverse arsenal of antimicrobial agents fails to conquer biofilms and intracellular Chlamydia. Likewise, even in long-term treatment with one antibiotic after another, infections persist. One of the primary problems is the inability of the antimicrobial agent to fully penetrate the biofilm leaving bacteria to exist in a protected state as they mutate and adopt a distinct and intrinsically resistant phenotype.

Many years ago someone wrote me who had a small infection at the base of their nail. This very quickly turned nasty and the patient's doctor thought it looked like gout. However, three weeks later the doctor changed his diagnosis to septicemia and wanted to go in and cut the finger open and possibly amputate. The patient refused and started applying iodine topically and taking it orally along with magnesium chloride transdermally. Within a few days the finger was less painful and less discolored. The swelling quickly went down and the normal healthy pinkness returned to the base of the finger.

NEW CANCER/FUNGUS THEORY

Cancer—always believed to be caused by genetic cell mutations—can in reality be caused by infections from viruses, bacteria, and fungi. "I believe that, conservatively, 15 to 20 percent of all cancer is caused by infections; however, the number could be larger—maybe double," said Dr. Andrew Dannenberg, director of the Cancer Center at New York-Presbyterian Hospital/Weill Cornell Medical Center. Dr. Dannenberg made the remarks in a speech in December 2007 at the annual international conference of the American Association for Cancer Research.

When the body's immune system weakens we get sick from one of a host of viruses, bacteria, and fungi that already live within us but are dormant. Change pH, oxygen, cell voltage, and hydration levels and these pathogens are ready to jump all over our blood streams and tissues. Cancer cells love the conditions that healthy cells abhor. Same goes for all infectious agents. It is impossible to be dying of cancer and not be dying of infections and nutritional deficiencies at the same time.

Science Daily said, "Infectious diseases are the world's number-one cause of death, with pathogenic fungi being responsible for extremely dangerous infections. Worldwide, more than €6 billion are spent each year on anti-fungal medications, and the total costs of the medical treatment of infectious diseases caused by pathogenic fungi are estimated in the order of hundreds of billions of Euros."

Over one million people worldwide are misdiagnosed with tuberculosis when in reality they have an incurable disease with a similar outlook to many cancers, says a recent report published in 2011 in the *Bulletin of the WHO*. The disease called "chronic pulmonary aspergillosis" (CPA) is a fungal infection not a bacterial infection. Is this incurable, totally drug-resistant TB infection fungal or bacterial? It looks very much like, or is identical to, TB when doctors look at it on a chest X-ray, and it has very similar symptoms initially. Doctors mistake it for TB and prescribe antibiotics as standard practice. Fifty percent of all patients who develop pulmonary aspergillosis are unlikely to survive for more than five years, a similar outlook to many cancers.

According to Dr. Milton White (specialty in internal medicine in Douglasville, Georgia), cancer is "neither the result of a virus nor the consequence of an inherited gene defect. Cancer is a hybrid. It is due to a plant bacterium (conidia) derived from an Ascomycete strain of fungus..."

Fungal Infections

According to *The Home Medical Encyclopedia*, in 1963, about 50 percent of all Americans suffered from an "unrecognized" systemic fungal infection. The cause of this infection has been attributed to several factors, some of which are antibiotics, birth control pills, excessive processed sugar and grain consumption, heavy metal contamination, xenoestrogens, alcohol, smoking, and chronic stress. These factors, combined with diets severely deficient in active enzymes and probiotics, have paved the way for one of the most prevalent fungal infections to date—*Candida albicans*.

In *Nature* we read, "Although viruses and bacteria grab more attention, fungi are the planet's biggest killers. Of all the pathogens tracked, fungi have caused more than 70 percent of the recorded global and regional extinctions, and now threaten amphibians, bats, and bees. The Irish potato famine in the 1840s showed just how devastating such pathogens are. Phytophthora infestans (an organism similar to and often grouped with fungi) wiped out as much as three-quarters of the potato crop in Ireland and led to the death of one million people."

Researchers estimate that there is 1.5 to 5 million species of fungi in the world, but only 100,000 have been identified. Reports of new types of fungal infection in plants and animals have risen nearly tenfold since 1995.

In 1999, Meinolf Karthaus, MD watched three different children with leukemia suddenly go into remission upon receiving a triple antifungal drug cocktail for their "secondary" fungal infections.

Fungi are dreadful enemies. During their life cycle fungi depend on other living beings, which must be exploited to different degrees for their feeding. Fungi can develop from the hyphae, the more or less beak-shaped specialized structures that allow the penetration of the host. The shape of a fungus is never defined; it is imposed by the environment in which the fungus develops. Fungi are capable of implementing an infinite number of modifications to their own metabolism in order to overcome the defense mechanism of the host. These modifications are implemented through plasmatic and biochemical actions as well as by a volumetric increase (hypertrophy) and numerical hyperplasia of the cells that have been attacked.

Doctors and Dentists at Fault

Dr. Elmer Cranton, author of *Bypassing Bypass*, says that, "Yeast overgrowth is partly iatrogenic (caused by the medical profession) and can be caused by antibiotics." Fungi (for example, *Aspergillus fumigatus*) are not affected by antibiotics and neither are viruses. If not given correct treatment (antifungal medication) the prognosis is that 50 percent of those infected will die inside 5 years. In fact, the overuse of antibiotics leads to fungal infections.

> When fungi become systemic from gut inflammation and the overuse of antibiotics, you can see how the whole body—again, the eyes, liver, gallbladder, muscles and joints, kidneys, and skin—becomes involved in inflammatory bowel disease.
> —Dr. Dave Holland

A new area of research being driven by Dundee life scientists is revealing remarkable abilities of fungi to interact with minerals and metals. Led by Professor Geoffrey Gadd in the College of Life Sciences, the research explores the unique taste that fungi seems to have for rock and heavy metal. This environmental science has demonstrated the incredible power of fungi, to eat through concrete and to absorb heavy metals, such as mercury and uranium in the environment.

Heavy metals create contaminated environments both inside and outside the cells. These environments attract all kinds of pathogens—viruses, bacteria, and fungi. Many cancers are caused by infections, which are themselves caused by heavy metal contamination. According to the observations made by the internationally recognized medical researcher, Dr. Yoshiaki Omura, all cancer cells have mercury in them. The single greatest source of mercury contamination is mercury containing dental amalgam and doctors around the world still inject children with mercury containing vaccines.

Each year in the U.S. an estimated 40 tons of mercury are used to prepare mercury-amalgam dental restorations. Scientific studies have concluded that the amalgam is the source for more than two-thirds of the mercury in our human population. On a daily basis, each amalgam releases on the order of 10 micrograms of mercury into the body. This mercury either accumulates in the body or is excreted via urine and feces into our wastewater systems.

Extreme Dangers

"Fungal infections cannot only be extremely contagious, but they also go hand in hand with leukemia—every oncologist knows this. And these infections are devastating: Once a child who has become a bone marrow transplant recipient gets a "secondary" fungal infection, his chances of living, despite all the anti-fungals in the world, are only 20 percent, at best," writes Dr. David Holland.

Doug A. Kaufman, author of *The Fungus Link* and host of the TV show *The Cause,* wrote:

> The day I wrote this, a young lady phoned into my syndicated radio talk show. Her three-year-old daughter was diagnosed last year with leukemia. She believes antifungal drugs and natural immune system therapy has been responsible for saving her daughter's life. She is now telling others with cancer about her daughter's case. After hearing her story, a friend of hers with bone cancer asked her doctor for a prescriptive antifungal drug. To her delight, this medication, meant to eradicate fungus, was also eradicating her cancer. She dared not share this with her physician, telling him only that the antifungal medication was for a "yeast" infection. When she could no longer get the antifungal medication, the cancer immediately grew back.

The Vitally Important P53 Gene

Along with phagocytosis (bodily defense mechanism), our p53 gene plays one of the most important roles in protecting us against cancer. It not only stops cancer invasion, but it also kills tumor cells, thereby preventing cancer from starting or getting out of control. However, in over 50 percent of all cancers, scientists have discovered that the patient's p53 gene was mutated and unable to stop cancer from initiating. According to the American Cancer Society, the p53 gene is the most studied of all genes because damage to this gene allows cells with damaged DNA, like cancer cells, to proliferate.

"Aflatoxin genotoxicity is associated with a defective DNA damage response bypassing p53 activation." This means that the mycotoxin, aflatoxin, found in our food supply, is capable of inactivating the p53 gene. The Proceedings of the National Academy of Science stated in 1993, that the mycotoxin, aflatoxin b1, made by Aspergillus fungus, is known to cause p53 mutations. Mycotoxins, made by fungi, are among the most carcinogenic substances known to science.

The Aspergillus mold toxin, aflatoxin B1, inhibits the breakdown of both glucose, or simple sugar, and glycogen. Fungi and the mycotoxins they produce impacts our genetic code, causing alterations that are found in a majority of cancers, reports Doug Kaufman. "Altering a cell's DNA amounts to changing the environmental code of that cell. Once changed the cell may respond differently—or not at all to outside hormones and enzymes that normally stimulate it to perform necessary functions. As one example of genetic alteration, aflatoxin B1 causes a break in DNA that alters the p53 tumor expression gene. Changes in this particular gene allow the cell to proliferate out of control. So it's no accident that this same mycotoxin can also go on to cause liver cancer"

Fungi are found in foods that we eat every day. Our primary concern is the long-term effects of ingesting food contaminated with low levels of mycotoxins," and that carcinogenic toxins, such as aflatoxin, a by-product of the Aspergillus molds, is a "common contaminant of peanuts, soybeans, grains, and cassava. It's a "frequent contaminant of wheat and corn." Without a properly functioning immune system, propped up and supported with significant iodine levels we're at risk of succumbing to various infectious and chronic diseases. Fungi invade our grain food supply because grains-a source of carbohydrates—are their favorite food.

VIRAL INFECTIONS ARE PH SENSITIVE

Viruses are extremely small parasitic life forms, the smallest living things on Earth. In essence, a virus is a minuscule pocket of protein that contains genetic material. Although viruses can remain dormant outside a living body, they only become active when in contact with live tissue. Once a virus infects a cell by penetrating the cell membrane, it can either lay dormant (lysogenic infection) or begin reproducing itself (lytic infection—the more common pattern). When a cell becomes full of virus, it bursts, releasing the virus to infect other host cells.

Certain viruses (including the rhinoviruses and coronaviruses that are most often responsible for the common cold and influenza viruses that produce flu) infect host cells by fusion with cellular membranes at low pH. Thus they are classified as "pH-dependent viruses."

As it is with viral infections, it is with cancer. The external pH of solid tumors is acidic as a consequence of increased metabolism of glucose and poor perfusion. Acid pH has been shown to stimulate tumor cell invasion and metastasis in vitro and in cells before tail vein injection in vivo.

Drugs that increase intracellular pH (alkalinity within the cell) have been shown to decrease infectivity of pH-dependent viruses. However pharmaceutical drugs that do this can provoke negative side effects. Sodium bicarbonate is the best way to increase pH in clinical emergency conditions and has been known as far back as the Spanish Flu pandemic of 1918 to save lives.

Increases of Carbon Dioxide and Bicarbonates
Lead to Increased Oxygen

The most important factor in creating proper pH is increasing oxygen because no wastes or toxins can leave the body without first combining with oxygen. The more alkaline you are, the more oxygen your fluids can hold and keep. Oxygen also buffers/oxidizes metabolic waste acids helping to keep you more alkaline. "The Secret of Life is both to feed and nourish the cells and let them flush their waste and toxins", according to Dr. Alexis Carrell, Nobel Prize recipient in 1912. Dr. Otto Warburg, also a Nobel Prize recipient, in 1931 and 1944, said, "If our internal environment was changed from an acidic oxygen deprived environment to an alkaline environment full of oxygen, viruses, bacteria, and fungus cannot live."

The position of the oxygen disassociation curve (ODC) is influenced directly by pH, core body temperature, and carbon dioxide pressure. According to Warburg, it is the increased amounts of carcinogens, toxicity, and pollution that cause cells to be unable to uptake oxygen efficiently. This is connected with over-acidity, which itself is created principally under low oxygen conditions.

According to Annelie Pompe, a prominent mountaineer and world-champion free diver, alkaline tissues can hold up to 20 times more oxygen than acidic ones. When our body cells and tissues are acidic (below pH of 6.5 to 7.0) they lose their ability to exchange oxygen, and cancer cells love that.

CONCLUSION

Iodine/iodide is the super medicine we need in the 21st century if we do not want to be slaughtered by infections as public health officials and medical scientists are promising. Iodine is just waiting, is already on the shelves, easily obtained on the Internet, and comes in many forms for many uses. Part 2 of the book, which follows, will provide a guide to using iodine, iodine product recommendations, and iodine dosages.

PART TWO
Guide to Using Iodine

5. Iodine and Chelation— Heavy Metals and Halogen Poisons

Heavy metals poison us by disrupting our cellular enzymes, which run on nutritional minerals, such as magnesium, zinc, and selenium. Toxic metals kick out the nutrients and bind their receptor sites, causing diffuse symptoms by affecting nerves, hormones, digestion, and immune function. The heavy metals most often implicated in human poisoning are lead, mercury, arsenic, and cadmium, but uranium is playing catch up since depleted uranium became the favorite armament of the United States military. Once in the body, they compete with and displace essential minerals and interfere with organ system function.

The Environmental Working Group has published a devastating report titled *Body Burden—The Pollution in Newborns.* "U.S. industries manufacture and import approximately 75,000 chemicals, 3,000 of them at over a million pounds per year. Studies show that hundreds of industrial chemicals circulate in the blood of a baby in the womb, interacting in ways that are not fully understood. Many more pollutants are likely present in the womb, but test methods have yet to be developed that would allow health officials to comprehensively assess prenatal exposure to chemicals, or to ensure that these exposures are safe. From a regulatory perspective, fetal exposure to industrial chemicals is quite literally out of control.

HEAVY METALS AND HALOGEN POISONS

Dr. Kellman of the Centre for Progressive Medicine in New York said, "Once damage to the thyroid takes place it affects all the other organs— starting with digestion and absorption. Toxins start accumulating in the system. You can have an array of symptoms: heart disease and its complications, high homocysteine levels, poor circulation, weight gain/loss, no appetite or bingeing, bloating, fluid retention, skin problems, aching joints, low blood pressure, high cholesterol, low libido, hair loss, and sensitivity to cold."

Iodine is the only option when it comes to removing these toxic haloids from the thyroid and even the pineal gland where fluoride concentrates, especially when there is a deficiency in iodine in the body. In an age of increasing radioactivity and toxic poisoning specifically with fluoride, chlorine, bromide, and mercury, iodine is a necessary mineral to protect us from harm for immediately these toxic substances will increasingly flow out of the body in the urine when high enough dosages of iodine are used.

Iodine intake immediately increases the excretion of bromide, fluoride, and some heavy metals, including mercury and lead. Bromide and fluoride are not removed by any other chelator or detoxifying technique.

Dr. Kenezy Gyula Korhaz of the Gyula Kenézy Hospital and Clinic in Budapest stated that iodine chelates heavy metals, such as mercury, lead, cadmium, aluminum, and halogens, such as fluoride and bromide, thus decreasing their iodine inhibiting effects, especially of the halogens. Iodine has the highest atomic weight of all the common halogens.

The mechanism of iodine in the cells is very ancient and lacking of specificity; cells are not able to distinguish iodide from other anions of similar atomic or molecular size, which may act as "pseudo-iodides": bromide, fluoride, chlorine, thiocyanate, cyanate, nitrate, pertechnate, and perchlorate.

Nowhere is this process more evident than in the case of the halides, which are all antagonistic elements to iodine, meaning they will impede the absorption of iodine. Heavy metals get stored in the same receptors that are looking for iodine. People who are exposed to bromine and fluorine are storing these toxic halides in iodine deficient receptors.

In the 1960s iodine added to bread increased the average daily intake 4 to 5 times RDA levels. Then they took the iodine out of the bread and some medical terrorist substituted bromide, a bio-poison in its place. There are actually four halogens: iodine, bromine, fluorine, and chlorine. All these halogens use the same receptors in the body. Therefore if a person's diet is deficient in iodine, the iodine receptors in the thyroid and stomach may fill up with bromine, which is common in grains, bleached flour, sodas, nuts, and oils as well as several plant foods. Iodine is depleted by bromine, which is used as a spray on fruits and vegetables, in baked goods, as a fumigant, and in Prozac, Paxil, and many other pharmaceutical drugs. Chlorine, fluorine, and fluoride are chemically related to iodine, and compete with it, blocking iodine receptors in the thyroid gland. Many of us are drinking fluoridated water and are brushing our teeth with fluoride toothpaste.

Dr. Donald Miller Jr. wrote, "There is growing evidence that Americans would have better health and a lower incidence of cancer and fibrocystic disease of the breast if they consumed more iodine. A decrease in iodine intake coupled with an increased consumption of competing halogens, fluoride, and bromide, has created an epidemic of iodine deficiency in America."

Fluoride

The human pineal gland contains the highest concentration of fluoride in the body. Fluoride is associated with depressed pineal melatonin synthesis and this depression increases one's chance of cancer. Any agent that affects pineal function could affect human health in a variety of ways, including effects on sexual maturation, calcium metabolism, parathyroid function, postmenopausal osteoporosis, and cancer.

Dr. David Brownstein says that fluoride inhibits the ability of the thyroid gland to concentrate iodine, and research has shown that fluoride is much more toxic to the body when there is iodine deficiency present. When iodine is supplemented the excretion rate of the toxic halides bromide, fluoride, and perchlorate is greatly enhanced. Brownstein says that after only one dose of iodine the excretion of fluoride increased by 78 percent, and this is very important for those who are drinking fluoridated water or are taking medicines with fluoride in them; bromide excretion rates increased by 50 percent.

Bromide and Chloride

Over the last three decades, bromine has contaminated our bread. Bromine blocks thyroid function and may interfere with the anticancer effect of iodine on the breast. Now, the risk for breast cancer is 1 in 8 and increasing 1 percent per year. Chlorine also blocks iodine in the body, so chlorinated water (both drinking and bathing) should best be avoided when possible. Iodine increases mobilization of bromine from storage sites with increased urinary excretion of bromide. Elevated bromide levels were observed in urine and serum samples, 20 times the levels reported in the literature in normal subjects.

*Patients who experience side effects while on orthoiodo-supplementation
are often excreting large amounts of bromide in the urine.*

Chloride competes with bromide at the renal level and increases the renal clearance of bromide thus, magnesium chloride is ideal for magnesium supplementation. Some patients require up to 2 years of iodine therapy to bring post loading urine bromide levels below 10 mg/24 hr., if chloride is not included in the bromine detoxification program. Rapid mobilization of bromine from storage sites with iodine supplementation combined with increased renal clearance of bromide with a chloride load often causes side effects. Increasing fluid intake and adding a complete nutritional program minimizes these side effects.

Dr. Guy E. Abraham noted that in some patients the excretion of lead, cadmium, and mercury increased several fold after only one day of iodine supplementation and that increased aluminum excretion was noted about a month after beginning supplementation. The symptoms of bromide include increased body odor and cloudy urine. The body odor lasts 1 to 2 weeks, but the cloudy urine may last several months before clearing up. Side effects can be minimized by increasing fluid intake. Increased fluid facilitates the excretion of excess iodine and the bromides, fluorides and heavy metals that the iodine displaces. Dr. Abraham also reported that the administration of magnesium in daily amounts up to 1200 mg eliminated the body odor but not the cloudy urine.

*Released bromide from storage sites can induce decreased
thyroid function, bromide being a potent goitrogen.*

Halogen Poisons

Iodine forms compounds with many elements, but is less reactive than the other members of its Group VII (halogens). There is a well-known law of halogen displacement. The critical activity of any one of these four halogens is in inverse proportion to its atomic weight. This means that any one of the four can displace the element with a higher atomic weight, but cannot displace an element with a lower atomic weight. For example, fluorine can displace chlorine, bromine, and iodine because fluorine has a lower atomic weight than the other three. Similarly, chlorine can displace bromine and iodine because they both have a higher atomic weight. A reverse order is not possible.

A knowledge of this chemical law brings us to the addition of chlorine to our drinking water as a purifying agent. Too many people are drinking water that is harmful to the body not because of its harmful germ content but because the chlorine content now causes the body to lose the much-needed iodine.

Chlorine Poisoning

Chlorine, which has been used extensively since 1904 to control microbes in public drinking water, belongs to the same class of elements as iodine; the "halogens" or elements that are one step removed from the "inert elements" (or gases) because they have just one electron missing from their outer shell to make it inert (non-reactive). This makes them quite readily reactive.

Chloride (Cl) is an essential element for humans, animals, and all plants. It is a component of common salt and found in seawater. The element exists in the plant soil system as the chloride anion Cl-. This must not be confused with other forms of the element, such as chlorine gas (highly toxic and unstable), chlorine in swimming pools, hypochlorite (a sterilant and bactericide), and hydrochloric acid (corrosive and dangerous liquid). The chlorine put in your water will slowly kill you where the chloride in magnesium chloride will nourish.

Cancer risk among people drinking chlorinated water is 93 percent higher than among those whose water does not contain chlorine.

—U.S. Council of Environmental Quality

Chloride is a prominent negatively charged ion of the blood, where it represents 70 percent of the body's total negative ion content. On average, an adult human body contains approximately 115 grams of chloride, making up about 0.15 percent of total body weight.

Chlorine is a dangerous gas that does not exist in the free elemental state in nature because of its reactivity, although it is widely distributed in combination with other elements. Chloride is a by-product of the reaction between chlorine and an electrolyte, such as potassium, magnesium, or sodium. Chloride salts are essential for sustaining human metabolism and have none of the effects of isolated chlorine gas.

Putting chlorine in the water supplies is a bad idea like putting bromide in bread. Cancer, heart trouble, premature senility are conditions attributable to chlorine treated water supplies. It is making us grow old before our time by producing symptoms of aging, such as hardening of the arteries.

Chlorine is a toxic gas that irritates the respiratory system. Always use care when opening a container of chlorine. Breathing in chlorine gas can knock you right out, and could be fatal.

Nothing can negate the incontrovertible fact, the basic cause of atherosclerosis and resulting entities, such as heart attacks and stroke, is chlorine.

—Dr. Joseph Price, author of *Coronaries/Cholesterol/Chlorine*

Iodine and Perchlorate Poisoning

The EPA's proposed safe exposure level for perchlorate is not protective of public health. CDC scientists have found that a significant number of women are at risk of thyroid hormone depression from perchlorate exposure. Perchlorate, the explosive ingredient in solid rocket fuel, has leaked from military bases and defense and aerospace contractors' plants in at least 22 states, is contaminating drinking water, dairy milk, produce and many other foods and plants affecting millions of Americans. CDC scientists have found that a significant number of women are at risk of thyroid hormone depression from perchlorate exposure. Perchlorate impairs the thyroid's ability to take up iodide and produce hormones critical to proper fetal and infant brain development. Further, studies show that breast milk may have even more worrisome levels of perchlorate.

The CDC/BU (Boston University) study, which examined breast milk from 49 Boston area women, found that the average breast fed infant in this study is being exposed to more than double the dose of perchlorate that the Environmental Protection Agency (EPA) considers safe; highly exposed babies are ingesting up to 10 times this amount.

In a related 2006 study, the CDC found perchlorate in the urine of every one of 2,820 people tested, suggesting that food is a key route of exposure in addition to drinking water. Applying the results of the CDC study to the California population, EWG estimates that at exposure to 5 ppb of perchlorate in drinking water, 1 in 10 California women of childbearing age with low iodine intake would be diagnosed as sub-clinically hypothyroid and require medical treatment when pregnant to protect themselves and their babies.

In the United States especially, people will want to note that iodine also is protective and effective at eliminating perchlorate from the body.

Iodine and Mercury Poisoning

Dr. Brownstein indicates that iodine is also a chelator of mercury and had tested quite carefully the amounts removed. Mercury not only poisons the nervous system and digestive tract, it can also poison the thyroid gland. There are 4 iodine binding sites or receptors on the thyroid gland. These receptors bind with the iodine we get from our diet. The iodine enters the thyroid and activates it. If the thyroid is not absorbing enough iodine it will not be fully activated and the body's temperature will be abnormally low. Mercury from dental fillings can migrate to the thyroid gland and sit on one or more of the thyroid's 4 iodine receptors blocking the iodine from reaching the receptors and activating the thyroid. When this happens iodine is not absorbed in normal amounts by the thyroid gland. The result is low body temperature or hypothyroidism.

Thanks to the continued promotion of mercury fillings by the American Dental Association and conventional dentists, consumers continue to be poisoned by this heavy metal that's placed into their mouths. There's so much mercury currently being put into the mouths of humans that the total volume of mercury being dumped into the environment from mercury fillings is nearly equal to that emitted by coal plants. Combine the two sources of mercury with a diet high in fish, which are contaminated with mercury and add a year's flu vaccine that also has mercury in it and we have a huge problem that health officials are not addressing at all.

MAGNESIUM DEFICIENCY

The involvement of free radicals in tissue injury induced by magnesium deficiency causes an accumulation of oxidative products in the heart, liver, kidney, skeletal muscle tissues, and in red blood cells. Magnesium is a crucial factor in the natural self-cleansing and detoxification responses of the body. It stimulates the sodium potassium pump on the cell wall, and this initiates the cleansing process in part because the sodium-potassium-ATPase pump regulates intracellular and extracellular potassium levels. "ATP production is essential for every cell to have an ample supply to deal with the challenges of metal overload, as it is required to even permit the cell to keep on pumping out calcium. Lack of ATP then is the underlying cause of abnormal calcification of tissues," writes Dr. Garry Gordon, known as the "father" of chelation therapy.

CHELATION THERAPY

Chelation therapy is a conventional treatment that involves the injecting of chemicals into the bloodstream to remove heavy metal and/or minerals (including mercury) that have built up in the body. One concern with traditional allopathic chelation therapy in general is that chelating agents are not as specific as we would like and are likely to remove essential trace minerals as well as toxic metals. Mercury drastically increases the excretion of magnesium and calcium from the kidneys. Both mercury itself and the drugs used to chelate mercury have a strong impact on mineral levels.

Limitations with the traditional allopathic chelation therapies include the fact that the agents used, while sometimes too specific to the metal targeted for removal, are also not protective enough when it comes to minerals that should be spared. Consequently essential trace minerals are likely to be depleted, making trace mineral replacement therapy absolutely essential. For example, EDTA (Ethylenediaminetetraacetic acid) is not effective for mercury, the number one toxic threat in most people. DMPS (2,3-dimercaptopropane-1-sulfonate) and DMSA (Dimercaptosuccinic acid) are dangerous to use because of their toxicity. Only highly trained physicians can safely administer them and even then we have problems like we do with most allopathic treatments.

No chelation or detoxification protocol can afford to ignore iodine.

Medical authorities warn of possible ill consequences to children undergoing chelation therapy. Along with metals, it is true that synthetic chelation also can strip the body of essential minerals like zinc and iron. In addition, as reported by doctors, the treatment can carry risks that include liver and kidney damage, bone-marrow problems, skin rashes, allergic reactions, and nutritional deficiencies. Medical authorities are correct in this regard for when chelation is done the allopathic way with synthetic drugs like DMPS, DMSA.

CONCLUSION

As you have learned in this section, iodine is unquestionably the best choice when it comes to removing toxic haloids and toxic heavy metals from the body. At a time of increasing radioactivity and toxic poisoning, iodine is a necessary mineral to protect us from their harm. The next chapter will provide you with iodine products that I recommend.

6. Iodine Product Recommendations

I continue to recommend liquid forms of iodine and selenium. For iodine, there is Nascent iodine for individuals and children affected by iodine and Lugol's for higher oral dosages and transdermal use. Moreover, for selenium I recommend Tung Oil, which is the only selenium safe for high dosages because it is bonded to a lipid.

The Nascent iodine is better for iodine sensitive individuals and for children where lower dosages are needed and recommended. Lugol's is less expensive for transdermal applications as well as higher oral dosages. When I take iodine orally, I also drop in a good amount of an exceptionally strong lipid based selenium called Tung Oil into the glass, even a small amount of selenium reduces the chances of dying of cancer by almost 50 percent. There are other products in solid form, but I have never used or recommended them.

Dr. Tina Kaczor writes, "Many of the iodine supplements on the market provide iodide (I-), usually potassium iodide, either alone or in combination with molecular iodine (I2). While this is safe for physiological repletion of iodine (doses less than 1,100 mcg/day), the salts carry greater risk of interfering with thyroid function at higher doses. The ideal supplement would contain molecular iodine with very little iodide. The difficulty is that iodine (I2) is rendered much more soluble with iodide (I-) and water (for example, Lugol's solution)."

There is documentation that doses 9 mg and higher may induce transient hypothyroidism as well as minor side effects, such as respiratory tract infection, headache, sinusitis, nausea, acne, diarrhea, rash, or abdominal pain. These side effects abated with the discontinuance of iodine, but it is important to realize that high-dose iodine is not without risk of side effects.

NASCENT IODINE

Nascent iodine, though more expensive, feels good while going down and is gentle enough to give to children, who do not seem to complain much about its taste. Nascent iodine contains approximately 400 mcg per drop, so 10 drops is 4 mg and 100 drops is only 40. It is safe to take much higher dosages than is suggested on the bottle. One has to ignore the suggested dosages on the bottle and take some of the information above as one's guidance for dealing with threatening radiation or deep iodine deficiencies that are more prevalent than doctors or the federal government will admit.

"An increasing number of my clients these days have some kind of issue with their thyroid. Many of them also have autoimmune disorders, parasites, *Candida,* and other sorts of unbalanced microbiomes. After working with Nascent iodine for over 3 years I have had enough amazing clinical results with Nascent iodine, that I recommend it for all my clients right away."

The Science Behind Nascent Iodine

Nascent iodine is a scientific term for iodine where the iodine molecule has the diatomic bond broken and has a high amount of electromagnetic energy associated with it. During the 2 to 3 hour of activation time (within the human body, once diluted in water and consumed) the Nascent iodine atom has the ability to be of assistance to the body. This atomic state and electromagnetic charge is held by the atom until diluted in water and consumed. Once diluted and inside the body this atom is readily absorbed and utilized by the body. This charged atom of iodine starts a process where it gradually loses its energy over 2 to 3 hours. During this time, the body recognizes this atom as the same iodine it produces in the thyroid in order to make the T3 and T4 hormones.

The atomic iodine is perhaps the least toxic and least irritating of all the iodine formulas available. The quality that separates Nascent iodine from all other iodine products is that the diatomic bond is broken with each atom keeping one of the two electrons that had made up the covalent bond. This is known as homolytic cleavage and causes the iodine atom to be subject to magnetic charging. The iodine being in the atomic state was the reason it was originally called Atomidine, for Atomic Iodine (1926 to 1935). This atomic state and large electromagnetic charge is held by the atom until diluted in water where it then rapidly loses its charge. Nascent iodine is a complete atom, no extra electrons, none missing.

It was the famous psychic Edgar Cayce, who suggested iodine for all sorts of thyroid problems, who advised that it would be necessary to electrically charge the iodine to change it into its "atomic" form. This charging converts the iodine into a form that the body can most fully recognize and assimilate. A true atomic iodine is the best kind to bring the thyroid to its optimal function because it supports and saturates the thyroid.

> *"Iodine has bactericidal activity, e.g. a 1 percent tincture will kill 90 percent of bacteria in 90 seconds, a 5 percent tincture in 60 second, and a 7 percent tincture in 15 seconds."*
> —Gershenfeld, 1968

Much of the information on iodine insists that iodine should be taken in its two major forms, iodide and iodine.

Iodine and Iodide

An iodide ion is an iodine atom with a -1 charge. Dr. David Brownstein wrote that, "It is very difficult to get iodine into a solution that uses water as a solvent. Therefore as Dr. Lugol discovered, using the reduced form of iodine (iodide) increases the solubility of iodine."

Atomic or Nascent iodine is not dissolved in water but in alcohol. Iodized salt and the iodine supplements usually found in health food stores contain the iodide form of iodine, but Dr. Brownstein has had little success treating patients with only iodide. The supplement Iodoral contains both the iodide (reduced) and iodine (oxidized) forms of iodine. The US RDA for iodine is 150 mcg. Iodoral contains 100 times (12.5 mgs) the RDAs requirement of iodine/iodide. One drop of Nascent iodine has 0.4 mg.

I do in fact find that when taking a Nascent form of iodine, therapeutic doses are lower. Most people will find that it is important to build up gradually in order to experience the least amount of detoxification reaction (see chapter on Iodine and Chelation). It is best when using strong chelators, which iodine is, to moderate the amount of detoxification symptoms or what is called the Herxheimer reaction, which is the experience of poisons being dumped into the blood stream from the cells or from large-scale yeast die offs.

Food that is present in the digestive tract will oxidize iodine to iodide, which is not corrosive to the gastrointestinal tract. Absorption is poor due to rapid conversion of iodine to iodide. This might explain why one needs to take very high doses of Iodoral or Lugol's compared to Nascent iodine, which seems to bypass the digestive track altogether meaning its absorption starts right in the mouth and continues through direct penetration of the stomach tissues. Iodide has to be converted back to the Nascent form in order to produce T3 and T4.

It is interesting to note that Salem Banajeh, Associate Professor-Child Health at Sana'a University-Sana'a-Yemen found that case fatality for malaria is 4 times higher in highlands compared with endemic areas. The further inland we go, the more populations are found to be iodine deficient.

Sunkar A. Bisey a Hindu scientist was suffering from malaria in the early nineteen-hundreds and quinine didn't do him any good. His life was in despair, and a Hindu doctor, hoping to save the life of India's greatest inventor, sent on a few doses of a Burmese preparation, made from seaweed, that had proved useful in treating chronic malaria there. Bisey tried it. The effect was electrical. He began to improve at once and in a month was a well man. He set out to research the contents of the seaweed and ended up producing the compound now known as Beslin or atomic iodine.

Malaria was treated with 20 drops of Nascent iodine in a half glass of water given 4 or 5 times during the first day and then going to 10 drops of Nascent iodine 4 times a day for 3 more days. A slide study of the blood shows that the malaria was gone from the body.

Dr. A. Regnault, while recognizing the great value of quinine in the treatment of malaria, said in 1901 that it was becoming a matter of general recognition that the quinine-series of drugs is of service only during certain developmental periods of the disease. It is held that the toxins are developed with great rapidity just at the time of the division of the parasites. In order to eliminate these toxins, Dr. Regnault suggested the use of iodine and potassium iodide.

LUGOL'S IODINE

Lugol's iodine solution is "old-fashioned" iodine. Lugol's iodine was first developed by the French physician, Jean Lugol, in 1829. It is a transparent brown liquid consisting of 10 parts potassium iodide (KI) to 5 parts iodine to 85 parts of (distilled) water. It is an effective bactericide and fungicide and, in fact, was, for the better part of a century, a common antiseptic—(though it has laboratory uses separate and apart from any medical application).

Dr. Lugol successfully treated many infectious conditions with this solution, which became known as Lugol's solution, and which is still available today without a prescription. Prior to World War II, many American and European physicians used Lugol's solution to treat thyroid conditions, using doses higher than 2 mg daily without apparent significant adverse effects.

In the U.S., Lugol's solution was previously unregulated and available over the counter as a general reagent, an antiseptic, a preservative, or as a medicament for human or veterinary application. However, effective August 1, 2007, the DEA now regulates Lugol's solution (all iodine solutions containing greater than 2.2 percent iodine) as a List I precursor because it may potentially be used in the illicit production of methamphetamine. By contrast, Lugol's iodine solution is available in the rest of the world at its original full strength formula.

I believe though Americans can still buy one bottle at a time legally, but many companies have already changed the formula so beware. Lugol's Solution 2 percent is simply a dilute formula of iodine and potassium iodide in water (2 percent iodine, 4 percent potassium iodide and 94 percent distilled water). You could just double (more or less) the use level to achieve the same dosage as the Lugol's Solution 5 percent. The formula ingredients are the same.

> WARNING: Do not take Lugol's iodine if you know you are allergic to iodine. If you know you are allergic try the Nascent iodine for it is rare to be allergic to this form. The Lugol's used to be a five percent solution of sodium iodine and 10 percent potassium iodide though companies now vary the original formula. Lugol's iodine has an optimal shelf-life of approximately one year though I have never seen a bottle of any type of iodine turn bad in this timeframe.

Following the Chernobyl nuclear reactor disaster in April, 1986, Lugol's iodine solution was administered to 10.5 million children and 7 million adults in Poland as a prophylactic measure against accumulation of radioactive iodine-131 in the thyroid.

Dr. David Brownstein commonly uses 50 mg and sometimes up to 100 mg to treat cancer and still does not notice toxic conditions. This makes sense because toxicity is on the gram not mg level. When I take it, which is almost every day, I do not bother to count the drops or measure the dosage, and I have never had a problem with iodine.

Potassium Iodide

Potassium iodide is a white crystalline salt with chemical formula KI, used in photography and radiation treatment. It finds widespread application as an iodide source because it is less hygroscopic than sodium iodide, making it easier to work with. KI can turn yellow upon heating in air or upon standing in moist air for long periods, because of oxidation of the iodide to iodine.

Potassium iodide was approved by the FDA in 1982 to protect the thyroid from radioactive iodine. In the event of an accident or attack at a nuclear power plant, or fallout from a nuclear bomb, several volatile fission product radionuclides may be released. Radioactive iodine is a common fission by-product and is particularly dangerous as the body concentrates it only in the thyroid gland which may lead to thyroid cancer. By saturating the body with a source of stable iodine prior to exposure, any radioactive iodine inhaled or ingested becomes the excess in the blood system and is excreted through the kidneys.

Dosages and Treatments

One drop of 5 percent Lugol's Iodine contains 6.417mg of elemental iodine. A 5-drop dose contains 32.09mg of elemental iodine. Lugol's iodine is a non-prescription item. Lugol's iodine solution in a 1 oz. dropper bottle. One oz. equals 576 drops.

An internal dosage of traditional Lugol's iodine was generally 1 or 2 drops in a glass of fruit juice, sipped throughout the course of a meal. This dosage depends on your body weight. As a guideline, if you weigh 60 kg or less the recommended amount is 1 drop, taken daily in a meal. If you weigh more than 60 kg, the recommended dose is 2 drops instead of one.

Dr. Hulda Clark (an alternative health practitioner) says, "Six drops of Lugol's solution can end it all for Salmonella. If you have gas and bloating, pour yourself 1/2 glass of water. Add 6 drops of Lugol's (not more, not less), stir with wood or plastic, and drink all at once. The action is noticeable in an hour. Take this dose 4 times a day, after meals and at bedtime, for 3 days in a row, then as needed. This eradicates even a stubborn case of Salmonella. Notice how calming 6 drops of Lugol's can be, soothing a manic stage and bringing a peaceful state where anxiety ruled before."

Retired biochemist and toxicologist Walter Last has this to say about Lugols: "Lugol's solution is an internal iodine solution designed to eliminate *Candida* and possibly viruses and other microbes from the bloodstream. Obtain 100ml of Lugol's solution, also labeled Aqueous Iodine Oral Solution B.P., from a chemist. Take a test drop in liquid other than just water to make it taste less strong. If this does not cause an allergic reaction, continue to take 4 times, 6 drops daily in liquid or mixed with food but not together with vitamins A, C, E, grape seed extract or cysteine. Iodine is an oxidant and it is best to reduce the intake of antioxidants while using it. If the blood was contaminated, then you may initially experience a die-off reaction of the *Candida*, causing weakness and possibly headache or nausea. If this happens, cut temporarily back on the amount of Lugol's solution and drink plenty of water and diluted teas or juices. Continue for 3 weeks, but interrupt if you develop a serious reaction. Do not take the iodine for more than 3 weeks, as that interferes with thyroid activity. If necessary repeat the course after several months."

Dr. J.C. Jarvis was particularly keen on the power of Lugol's iodine, for treating various illnesses, including colds and flu, and for countering the effects of stress: "Supposing you do follow the suggestions outlined above and find that some weeks the pressures of your private and your business life are causing you to lose the ability to bounce back. Then you should add a drop of Lugol's solution of iodine to your glass of apple or grape juice at breakfast or you may take it in the mixture of apple cider vinegar and water. The point is that the potassium in the solution (Lugol's is 10 percent potassium iodide) blocks off the body mechanism that organizes for aggressive action, releasing its hold on the body when opportunity for rest and relaxation arises. The iodine swings into action the body and the building up and storing of body reserves. When working under pressure, include the Lugol's solution dose each day until the period of pressure passes. If it should happen that your body becomes saturated with iodine, you will find that there is an increase of moisture in the nose. If this occurs, omit the iodine until the nose is normal."

IODINE AND INSTANT WATER PURIFICATION

Iodine is a very effective method for water purification. Its action is dependent on the concentration of iodine, the water temperature, and duration of contact. For example, a concentration of 8 mgs per liter at 20 degrees centigrade will destroy all pathogens if left for 10 minutes. Lower concentrations and lower water temperatures require a longer duration of action.

Iodine tablets were developed during World War II to disinfect small amounts of water for emergency or temporary use. A few drops of tincture of iodine or iodine tablets are popular with campers and the military for disinfecting water. An iodine residual of 0.5 to 1.0 mg/l should be maintained, and iodine at this level gives the water little or no iodide taste or odor.

Today one can harness the power of iodine in the LifeStraw, a personal, portable water purifier that eliminates virtually all waterborne bacteria and most viruses responsible for causing diarrheal diseases. The LifeStraw, introduced in 2005, is 10 inches long and weighs about 4.3 ounces. When someone sucks through the straw, the water flows through textile and iodine filters, which kill off bacteria, such as E. coli and viruses. A second chamber consists of granulated active carbon that absorbs residual iodine, thereby improving the taste of the water.

One straw is capable of purifying at least 700 liters (182 gallons) of water, removing an estimated 99.9 percent of bacteria and 99 percent of waterborne viruses. The straw doesn't completely remove turbidity from water or make saline water potable. It also doesn't remove or filter heavy metals. The product, which costs as little as $3, has won a number of awards, including the 2008 Saatchi & Saatchi Award for World Changing Ideas. LifeStraw has the potential to save many lives.

"The LifeStraw empowers people so they don't have to wait for the government to come up with solutions," says Mr. Frandsen, who is now 36 and president and chief executive officer of the family's Lausanne, Switzerland-based company, Vestergaard Frandsen, which manufactures the LifeStraw. The light blue straw with a resilient polystyrene shell should be on everyone's survival list as we prepare for the increasing difficulties in the world.

Relief agencies are using this straw for communities
devastated by natural disasters.

Jeff Nene, a spokesman for Convoy of Hope, says people in dire situations make the mistake of drinking dirty water, not realizing the impurities can cause diarrhea, dysentery, and eventually death. "You can go for a long time without food," he says. "But you can't live long without water."

CONCLUSION

Most believe that Lugol's iodine solution is a safe and effective way to provide adequate amounts of iodine for proper thyroid hormone production, responsible for our metabolic rate, normal growth and development, protein, carbohydrate, and fat metabolism amongst other things. Lugol's is certainly ideal for transdermal use. Though the Nascent iodine is much more efficient, it is expensive if one is interested in taking iodine levels up to their upper limits. Even with today's less concentrated Lugol's solutions, they are still considerably more concentrated thus more appropriate than Nascent for transdermal usage. Small bottles of higher concentration are still legally available. The next chapter will provide more on ideal iodine dosages and the transdermal use of iodine.

7. *Iodine Dosages and Applications*

Iodine is necessary for the proper function of many of the body's tissues, including the breasts, pancreas, brain, stomach, adrenal glands, skin, salivary glands, and cerebral spinal fluid. Iodine deficiency can lead to a dysfunction of these tissues and cause a number of symptoms, see page 30. Some studies have shown that iodine deficiency leads to a higher risk of developing various cancers, especially of the breast, prostate, and ovaries. Do not wait for any of these conditions to arrive, everyone today will benefit from higher iodine intake.

Humans tolerate large doses of iodine. The ultra-high doses that were used a century ago are helpful in medical emergencies—specifically when facing antibiotic resistant infections, viruses, and stubborn fungal and yeast infections. Iodine's true role—making up more than 1/2 of the body's immune system—is not well understood. Deficiencies in iodine have a great effect on the immune system and its response to infectious diseases including cancer, which in many cases, up to 40 percent, are caused by infections.

The National Health and Nutrition Survey undertaken by the CDC showed iodine levels falling over 50 percent in the last 30 years. In 1940, the average American got 800 micrograms of iodine in their diet. In 1995 we averaged 135 micrograms, an 83 percent decline! The Japanese consume 89 times more iodine than Americans, due to their daily consumption of sea vegetables, and they have reduced rates of many chronic diseases, including the lowest rates of cancer in the world. Why do medical organizations and the medical press promote everything but iodine for the treatment and prevention of cancer?

Even at low dosages, iodine is a powerhouse. So effective is iodine that aerosols can be effective in sterilizing a room at levels not even detectable by humans. However, Dr. David Derry says, "Dietary iodine found in iodized salt is below the amounts needed to fill mucus defense roles. To protect themselves, people wishing to boost their defense against infections should use an iodine supplement in their diets. Why would people need the larger doses of iodine? Why have iodine levels fallen 50 percent in the last 30 years? As I pondered these questions, I came to the conclusion that the toxicity of modern life must be impacting iodine levels. It is well known that the toxic halides, fluoride, and bromide, having a similar structure as iodine, can competitively inhibit iodine absorption and binding in the body. Because of the elevated levels of toxic halides in the environment and in the food supply, iodine levels have not only fallen but larger amounts of iodine are necessary to correct iodine deficiency as well as to promote a detoxifying effect of heavy metals."

When treating life-threatening diseases we do not have months to fool around with low dosages. The anti-microbial process of iodine quickly kills bacteria, viruses, fungi, and various other microorganisms if a high enough dosage is used. We need to dial up iodine levels quickly when we use it to fight infections. Iodine can be taken internally in large quantities and will have the same effect internally as it does on external surfaces. In addition, as in breast cancer, we often need to get it concentrated to certain tissues or organs, and we do that by painting the breasts with iodine.

IODINE DOSAGES IN THE PAST

Just to give you an idea of how high iodine dosages have been taken to in the past we have to revisit the 1930s when iodine was still a universal medicine, listed in the U.S. Pharmacopeia and was used at much higher dosages than anyone even dreams of using today. The usual dose for treatment was 300 mgs (46 drops of full strength Lugol's) to 1 gm (1000 mg, 154 drops).

"Extremely high doses of iodine can have serious side effects, but only a small fraction of such extreme doses are necessary to kill influenza viruses," continues Derry who tells us, "In 1945, a breakthrough occurred when J.D. Stone and Sir McFarland Burnet (who later went on to win a Nobel Prize for his Clonal Selection Theory) exposed mice to lethal effects of influenza viral mists. The lethal disease was prevented by putting iodine solution on mice snouts just prior to placing them in chambers containing influenza viruses."

Dr. Gabriel Cousens wrote, "Recently Dr. Mercola [alternative medicine expert and osteopathic physician] surprisingly stated that the highest amount of daily iodine intake should be no more than 400 micrograms. This is only slightly higher than the FDA recommendation, which is 150 to

290 micrograms daily, dependent upon age, gender, and life cycle. However, it is dramatically less than what some of the leading iodine medical experts suggest, as closer to, at least, 12 to 18 milligrams daily, approximately 45 times higher. Why this discrepancy? And how can Dr. Mercola, who is often so correct in his understanding, in my opinion, miss the mark exponentially?"

Cousens states, "Historically, as early as 1911, (11th edition of the 1910 to 1911 Encyclopedia Britannica) people normally took between 300,000 to 900,000 micrograms daily without incident. This is over 2,000 times more than Dr. Mercola's recommendation. How is it that now only 1/5,000th of this dose is now considered safe? In 1948, there was a poorly performed and, since then, never replicated study alleging what is known as the Wolff-Chaikoff effect, [see page 29]. The Wolff-Chaikoff effect suggested that theoretically hypothyroidism could occur as a result of excess iodine. This study indicated a decreased dosage to 2 milligrams daily would be safer. (This is still an amount 5 times higher than what Dr. Mercola is recommending.) Even the Food and Nutritional Board at the Institute of Medicine has set the tolerable upper limit of 1,100 micrograms of iodine daily (3 times higher than Dr. Mercola's recommendation). Other researchers have used between 3,000 and 6,000 micrograms/day to prevent goiter (14 times higher than Dr. Mercola's recommendation). Iodine is found in every single one of our body's hundred trillion cells. Without adequate iodine levels life is impossible. Iodine is the universal health nutrient and brings health on many levels."

IODINE DOSAGES TODAY

The current U.S. daily recommended allowance (RDA) for iodine is set at 150 mcg for non-pregnant adults. Dr. Michael B. Schachter, certified in psychiatry and nutrition, says, "The treatment dose when a person is iodine insufficient is generally between 12.5 mg and 50 mg daily. Preliminary research indicates that if a person is iodine insufficient, it takes about three months to become iodine sufficient while ingesting a dosage of 50 mg of iodine daily and a year to achieve that while ingesting a dosage of 12.5 mg of iodine daily.

For those who are interested in maintained dosages after disease and deficiencies have been dealt with understand that your thyroid gland alone needs about 6 mg of iodine per day for optimal function; the breasts of a woman will need approximately 5 mg/day (women with larger breasts need more); and other body tissues such as your adrenal glands, thymus, ovaries, hypothalamus, and pituitary gland need about 2 mg/day. Thus for optimal wellness, adults should consider approximately 10 to 12 mg/day.

One of my neighbors, who had cancer, visited the Gerson Clinic in Mexico and came back with a protocol suggesting one drop of Lugol's a day. I of course have him taking much more. When I take, I do not count the drops. Easier and more efficient to just use a drop or two though there are iodine sensitive people who need to be extremely cautious about dosages, especially when just starting iodine supplementation.

Dr. David Brownstein said, "After testing individuals and finding low iodine levels, I began to use smaller milligram amounts of iodine/iodide (6.25 mg/day). Upon retesting these individuals 1 to 2 months later, little progress was made. I therefore began using higher milligram doses (6.25 to 50 mg) to increase the serum levels of iodine. It was only with these higher doses that I began to see clinical improvement as well as positive changes in the laboratory tests." Brownstein has sometimes used between 200 and 300 milligrams of iodine daily, with higher doses for more serious and difficult diseases.

"At 6 grams daily (which is 6 million micrograms/day or 6,000 milligrams/day!), a much higher dose, iodine has been used to cure syphilis, skin lesions, and chronic lung disease," says Cousens. "From a larger physiological perspective, it is important to realize that the thyroid is only one gland of many glands and tissues that needs iodine. Other glands/organs/systems with high iodine uptake are the breasts, ovaries, cervix, blood, lymph, bones, gastric mucosal, salivary, adrenal, prostate, colon, thymus, lungs, bladder, kidney, and skin. Iodine is found and used in every hormonal receptor in the body."

Dr. Jorge Flechas, a specialist in iodine therapy for thyroid disorders, has found in a study that iodine can reduce the need for insulin in diabetic patients, using 50 to 100 mg of iodine per day. Of 12 patients, 6 were able to completely come off their medications with random glucose readings below 100 mg/dl and a HbA1c less than 5.8 (normal), and the other 6 were able to reduce the amount and/or number of medications needed to control their diabetes.

Gradual Dose Buildup

Many people will discover that it is important to build up gradually in order to experience the least amount of detoxification reaction from taking iodine. Ideally use strong chelators, which iodine is, to moderate the amount of detoxification symptoms or what is called the Herxheimer reaction (see page 65). This is most readily controlled with iodine in the Nascent atomic form simply because it is so easy to control and regulate low dosages.

Supplementing with iodine can replenish your iodine stores while flushing out poisons. People usually do not experience the negative effects of some type of detoxification when using iodine unless they are removing unusually high levels of bromide and fluoride. Most people actually notice increased energy, better sleep, and mental clarity. Over the last 30 years, our iodine intake has declined 50 percent, while the ingestion of toxic competing halogens (bromine, fluorine, chlorine, and perchlorate) has dramatically increased.

Iodine sensitive and thyroid compromised patients should read Dr. David Brownstein's book, *Iodine: Why You Need It, Why You Can't Live Without It*, on iodine and thyroid conditions. Many people are already severely thyroid compromised and are on drugs that complicate things.

Bottom Line

Without iodine to control infection and surgery, hospitals in general become inherently more dangerous. For that matter, in the future, without iodine, no one would go into a hospital unless they absolutely had to because of all the germs on floors and other surfaces and floating around in the air, and nothing the doctors will give in terms of antibiotics will help because they have already created so many antibiotic resistant strains of pathogens.

The last thing we need to be afraid of is iodine used in high enough dosages to take down infections that are life-threatening (see the inset on page 76). Do not be shy about administering high dosages unless it is the first administration of iodine to a thyroid-compromised patient. That said, if there is time, always start out with low dosages. It is like putting your toe in hot water to see if you can get safely into the tub. Check out your sensitivity to iodine if you are a first time user.

TRANSDERMAL IODINE

Surgeons scrub with iodine and they have their nurse paint iodine on their patients because the tincture of iodine remains the best antiseptic for preventing wound infections after surgery. Iodine has a long illustrious history as the following story presented by Dr. Derry illustrates. It is the most legendary of documentations of transdermal iodine therapy applied to a famous person in the American Civil War:

> On September 29, 1862, Colonel John B. Gordon held the center of General Lee's army at the battle of Antietam or Sharpsburg. The

Iodine Toxicity

The human body is in need of iodine, but there is a limit. Severe iodine poisoning is rare and generally occurs only when taking large megadoses, doses of many grams, to cure disease or to detox from chemical exposure.

Dr. David Brownstein, in his book, *Iodine: Why You Need It; Why You Can't Live Without It,* says, "Of all the elements known so far to be essential for human health, iodine is the most misunderstood and the most feared. Yet, iodine is the safest of all the essential trace elements, being the only one that can be administered safely for long periods of time to large numbers of patients in daily amounts as high as 100,000 times the RDA. However, this safety record only applies to inorganic, non-radioactive forms of iodine. Some organic iodine containing drugs are extremely toxic and prescribed by physicians. The severe side effects of these drugs are blamed on inorganic iodine although studies have clearly demonstrated that it is the whole molecule that is toxic, not the iodine released from it."

In treating over 4,000 patients, Dr. Brownstein has found only 3 patients with "allergy" to non-radioactive inorganic iodine/iodide. The Nascent form (*see* page 64) is even less provoking meaning the chances of side effects besides a normal detoxification and chelation response would be near zero.

Excess iodine has symptoms similar to those of iodine deficiency. Commonly encountered symptoms are abnormal growth of the thyroid gland and disorders in functioning and growth of the organism as a whole. Acute iodine toxicity is rare, however when iodine is taken in large doses symptoms may include abdominal pain, burning of the mouth and throat, fever, nausea, vomiting, diarrhea, and a weak pulse. Iodine is a poison if taken in larger amounts; if 2 to 3 grams of it is consumed, it could be fatal.

Dr. Abraham started his Iodine Project around 1998 when he became aware of the many benefits of treating patients with iodine using doses far beyond the 2 mg a day, which most physicians consider to be poten- tially toxic. He noted that starting in the 1820s, the French physician Jean Lugol used these higher doses to treat a wide variety of conditions.

first volley from the northern lines sent a ball through the calf of Gordon's right leg; soon after, another went through the muscles of his thigh; a third pierced his left arm, tearing asunder the tendons and mangling the flesh; a forth ripped through his shoulder leaving a wad of clothing embedded in its track. Still, no bones were broken; but, while Gordon lingered in the firing line, "with," as he says himself, "but little of my usual strength," a fifth ball struck him squarely in the face.

Dr. Weatherly of the 6th Alabama Regiment, in charge of medical arrangements, had the Colonel removed to a base hospital, and prescribed tincture of iodine to be painted on the wounds three or four times a day. The case was unpromising. Gordon's eyelids were greatly swollen; one eye was completely closed, the other almost so; his jaw was immovably clenched, and, to make matters worse, erysipelas (staphylococcus infection of skin) had set in on the left arm.

Mrs. Gordon, his wife, who nursed him—her name was Fanny, and was then a beautiful girl of 25—put a liberal interpretation on her instructions and painted the wounds, not three or four times a day, but, as Gordon himself says: "I think three to four hundred times a day." Fanny's diligence and devotion were rewarded. Her husband survived, outlived the war, and became the Governor of Georgia, a General, and Commander-in-Chief of the United Confederate Veterans. He died in 1904.

Dr. Abraham writes, "The bioavailability of iodine applied to the skin is well known. Over 100 years ago, application of iodine to the skin was used extensively for iodine supplementation." In 1932, Nyiri and Jannitti from the College of Pharmacy of Rutgers University wrote, "Iodine is being used extensively as a prophylactic and therapeutic agent by application to the outer integument, (the skin) and has maintained its place in medicine for many decades."

Dr. Derry says, "Iodine put onto scabs helps to organize total repair of the tissue. All pre-malignant lesions and many other oddities of the skin appear to respond to this regeneration process triggered by topical iodine. I have mentioned previously a patient with a biopsy-proven breast cancer lesion (she refused surgery because of previous cancer treatment) that was strongly fixed to the skin responding well to topical iodine and ended up being a dimple on the breast 3 years later. It is my belief a water solution of iodine (like Lugol's) is an important therapeutic agent for skin. Because of its effectiveness and the results, perhaps many skin diseases are related to local tissue areas of relative iodine deficiency. In addition, iodine's ability to trigger natural cell death (apoptosis) makes it effective against all pre-cancerous skin lesions and likely many cancerous lesions."

Painting Iodine on my wrist gets rid of my sore throat every time! Iodine definitely works for me, however, I find it best to use the clear "decolorized" iodine, available at most drugstores. I paint it on the inside of the wrists (where the veins are closest to the skin) and on the sides of the throat.

In her testimonial, Claire W. states:

I get small lesions on my forearms and the backs of my hands which I've been told by a doctor could become cancerous. In the past, I have had that doctor "burn off" these spots with nitrogen. That has usually worked, but did not work on two areas that have been with me for about 3 years now. For a while now I've been painting these areas with Lugol's solution (5 percent iodine), only three or four times a week as the iodine does not absorb as it would elsewhere on the skin and the dark red/brown of the iodine is very noticeable. These lesions are not completely gone yet, but they are definitely fading away.

"Iodine sprayed on the mucous lining of a woman's vagina will be absorbed and will soften her breasts in a matter of 5 minutes, while at the same time it relieves the tension and irritability of intestinal musculature," writes Dr. John Myers.

Iodine is an antiseptic and can be used to kill bacteria and fungi. Iodine used topically as a douche is effective against a wide range of organisms, including candida and chlamydia.

—Dr. David Brownstein

Povidone iodine (topical use only), also known as iodopovidone, is an antiseptic utilized for skin disinfection before and after surgery. It has been used for:

- Cataract surgery antisepsis: 1 percent povidone-iodine solution used preoperatively

- Chronic otitis media: 5 percent povidone-iodine ear drops, 3 drops taken three times daily for 10 days has been used

- Upper airway sterilization: 1 percent povidone-iodine solution inhaled via nebulizer twice daily has been used, with gargle twice daily

It should be noted that povidone iodine contains surfactant (reduces the surface tension of a liquid) and sticking agents (polymers) making it more toxic/dangerous to use than other iodine.

IODINE DOUCHES

Routine douching is not necessary to maintain vaginal hygiene; the preponderance of evidence suggests that douching may be harmful and shows an association between douching and numerous adverse outcomes. Povidone iodine is not ideal for internal use and cannot be compared at all to atomic (nascent) forms of iodine.

> *Douche preparations containing povidone iodine are widely used,*
> *and efforts have been made to treat and/or prevent*
> *vaginal infections with povidone iodine.*
>
> —Dr. David Brownstein

However, in 1997, Zhang and colleagues reported the results of a meta-analysis of six studies of vaginal douching and cervical cancer. Four studies were conducted in the United States and published in 1979, 1986, 1987, and 1991; two in Latin America were published in 1990 and 1995. The combined results suggest an overall positive effect.

Douche and vaginal suppositories containing 10 percent PVP-Iodine (Providone-iodine) have been reported effective in the treatment of vaginal infections. These can be used both as a topical and therapeutic agent for the treatment of birth-canal infections and for various forms of vaginitis. PVP-Iodine has been reported as a very effective bactericide against organisms commonly found in the mouth and is able to destroy these within 15 seconds. Using a mouthwash/gargle product containing 0.5 percent PVP-Iodine is effective in reducing the bacterial flora in the mouth prior to dental surgery.

I use Lugol solution for iodine, either 6 drops in water or sometimes I put it directly on my skin. If it absorbs within a short period of time [hours] I know that I am deficient so I put it on every couple of hours until I get to the point of a 24-hour lapse when the color is still remaining on the skin—which is supposed to mean that my body has enough. But, I find taking the drops a lot less bothersome and easier to remember.

—Nancy G.

Dr. Daniel H. Duffy said, "I have been using IODEX, an iodine containing paste applied directly to the skin for the past 32 years to help break up the intercostal pain and palpatory soreness at the sternum often suffered by a high percentage of Midwesterners, especially female hypothyroids. I was also taught early on that it was common practice for veterinarians to rub IODEX on the fetlocks of horses to eliminate cystic formations. Women are instructed to rub IODEX into the sore spots at the intercostals [muscles] at bedtime until the soreness disappears."

IODINE PREPARATIONS

Iodine preparations include aerosol sprays, gauze pads, lubricating gels, creams, solutions, douche preparations, suppositories, gargles, perineal wash solutions, shampoos, and skin cleansers and scrubs.

Lugol's iodine tincture usually contains 2 percent iodine and 2.4 percent sodium iodide (NaI) dissolved in 50 percent ethanol; it is used as a skin disinfectant. Strong iodine tincture contains 7 percent iodine and 5 percent potassium iodide (KI) dissolved in 95 percent ethanol; it is more potent but also more irritating than tincture of iodine. Iodine solution contains 2 percent iodine and 2.4 percent NaI dissolved in aqueous solution; it is used as a non-irritant antiseptic on wounds and abrasions. Strong iodine solution (Lugol's solution) contains 5 percent iodine and 10 percent KI in aqueous solution.

Iodophores (such as, povidone-iodine) are water-soluble combinations of iodine with detergents, wetting agents that are solubilizers, and other carriers. They slowly release iodine as an antimicrobial agent and are widely used as skin disinfectants, particularly before surgery. Povidone iodine preparations are applied topically to the skin and to membranes, for example, vaginal membranes, and in infected wounds and surgical incisions. The uses continue to be largely medicinal though used in industrial sanitation and disinfection in hospitals, building maintenance, and food-processing operations.

Povidone Iodine

The use of conventional povidone iodine, such as compositions, which have a povidone to iodine ratio of fewer than 10 to 1, typically 8.5 to 1, in vaginal treatments, has been reported. Women being prepared for total abdominal hysterectomy were treated by insertion of povidone-iodine tampons that remained in the vagina until the end of the operation. Statistically significant decreases both in infectious morbidity and in the percentage of positive cultures from the cervix and vagina, at the time of the operation resulted from this use of povidone-iodine.

The use of povidone-iodine ('Betadine') pessaries in the treatment of candidal and trichomonal vaginitis was reported by a Dr. Henderson. He studied one hundred and thirty-five women suffering from trichomonal, candidal, or both infections simultaneously, and were treated with povidone-iodine pessaries, 2 pessaries being inserted nightly. The results obtained were very encouraging, 92 percent of the trichomonal and 96 percent of the candidal infections would be cured if treatments were continued for a month. Short treatments of only 7 days were not effective.

Topical Iodine

The best iodine for transdermal use is the 7 percent iodine, but as of August 1, 2007 it became a controlled substance regulated by the Drug Enforcement Administration (DEA) under the chemical regulatory provisions of the Controlled Substances Act (CSA). The DEA believes that this action is necessary to remove deficiencies in the existing regulatory controls, which have been exploited by drug traffickers who divert iodine (in the form of iodine crystals and iodine tincture) for the illicit production of methamphetamine in clandestine drug laboratories. One can only purchase small bottles of the 7 percent solution. Weaker solutions will work, but much more of it needs to be used. Many studies for transdermal use have been done with PVP-Iodine, which is appropriate for external uses only. The inexpensive tinctures available in drug stores are also for external use only.

It is important when considering using iodine transdermally to take into account the large amount lost by evaporation. The evaporation of iodine from the skin increases with increased ambient temperatures and decreased atmospheric pressure due to weather conditions and altitude. For example, the yellow color of iodine will disappear much faster in Denver, Colorado at 5,000 feet above sea level then Los Angeles, California at sea level, irrespective of the amount of bioavailability of iodine. For this reason, Dr. Simoncini directs skin cancer patients to paint the iodine on 20 times.

To summarize Dr. Guy E. Abraham's findings:

- Free iodine penetrates through the unbroken skin.

- Approximately 88 per cent of the iodine evaporates from the surface within 3 days.

- Colloidal iodine evaporates somewhat more quickly than tincture of iodine; Lugol's solution is more stable than either of them.

- The influence of ambient temperature on the evaporation of iodine is significant: within the first minute, the losses of iodine by evaporation are: 10 to 15 percent at 9 c; 18 to 25 percent at 24 c; and 35 percent at 37c.

- The remaining iodine on the skin following evaporation of 88 percent of the total iodine, approximately 12 percent, is at the disposal of the body, and penetrates through the skin. The bioavailability of the remaining 12 percent of the skin iodine is very gradual.

Regeneration of Human Scar Tissue with Topical Iodine

Dr. David M. Derry talks about using Lugol's iodine to regenerate human scar tissue. He says, "Regeneration starts a few days after applying iodine and stops and forms adult scar if applications are discontinued. One face scar has completely regenerated. The hypothesis that topical iodine in the form of Lugol's solution regenerates human scar tissue back to normal is supported by preliminary findings."

PRINCIPLES AND PRACTICES OF TRANSDERMAL MEDICINE

Iodine can be used as a principle agent in the treatment of cancer with specific attention paid to breast and skin cancer, which are most easily treated transdermally. It is useful to know that in the case of iodine (magnesium as well) transdermally does not mean just topically, it also includes aerosol (direct application to the lungs) as well as for the upper and lower ends of the GI track, (colonics and oral use for treatment of oral and stomach cancers) as well as in douches for cancers of cervix and uterus.

Transdermal medicine delivers medications to the exact site of injury/pain.

One of the principle reasons iodine is so effective for skin cancer is that, according to Dr. Simoncini, a physician and alternative medicine advocate, skin cancers are caused by *Candida* fungus, which has adapted itself to metabolizing the most proteinaceous constituents of the epidermis. Dr. Simoncini perhaps has the most experience with transdermal iodine in cancer treatment, but even he did not realize that you can treat internal cancers through raising internal iodine concentrations through oral administration.

Iodine, when applied to the breasts or any other part of the body can cause the skin to become dry and leathery. Sometimes red lines appear looking like bloodshot Halloween eyeballs. In such cases stop the transdermal iodine application and wait for the skin to return to normal and then try again with lighter and less frequent application. Or as soon as one sees irritation or skin burn use a CBD (cannabidiol) topical salve or an excellent product called Relief Rx. After iodine dries, the woman or her attending companion or nurse could tenderly apply a topical cannabinoid salve/cream (regular medical marijuana or CBD, which is marijuana without THC) to the breasts, thus soaking them with all of marijuana's anti-cancer effects.

Other topical treatments to the breasts can and should include magnesium oil massaged into the breasts, clay packs, slow breathing, and even infrared treatments. In the future, we will see sound waves used to heat the tissues to the point where cancer cells cannot survive, but normal healthy cells do. Every cancer patient should be using sodium bicarbonate to alkalinize his or her tissues.

Transdermal medicine is ideal for pain management as well as sports and pediatric medicine. In fact it is one of the best ways of administering medicines quickly and effectively. Transdermal methods of delivery are widely used because they allow the absorption of medicine directly through the skin. Gels, emulsion creams, sprays, and lip balm stick applicators are easy to use and are effective in getting medicine into the blood stream quickly. Iodine used transdermally is a good idea and has been used so for over a hundred and fifty years.

Traditional methods of administering medicine, such as tablets or capsules, get watered down and become much less effective due to stomach acids and digestive enzymes, before they eventually get into the bloodstream. Bypassing the stomach and liver means a much greater percentage of the active ingredient goes straight into the bloodstream where it's needed. In many cases, transdermal methods are used to help avoid potential side effects, such as stomach upset or drowsiness.

Drugs enter different layers of skin via intramuscular, subcutaneous, or transdermal delivery methods. The most common ways to administer drugs are oral (swallowing an aspirin tablet), intramuscular (getting a flu shot in an arm muscle), subcutaneous (injecting insulin just under the skin), intravenous (receiving chemotherapy through a vein), or transdermal (by wearing a skin patch). It is not a surprise, when you consider the large surface area of the skin, that when you apply a substance to the entire body, rapid absorption and resultant effect is sufficient to put transdermal administration on par with other ways of administering drugs.

Transdermal medicine is a versatile form of medicine everyone can use and benefit from. With transdermal medicine we can address systemic nutritional deficiencies, act to improve immune, hormonal, and nervous systems, protect cells from oxidative damage, open up cell wall permeability, reduce the risk of cancers, shrink tumors, and do just about anything else we do with oral and intravenous drugs.

ABSORPTION

Medicines can enter the body in many different ways, and they are absorbed when they travel from the site of administration into the body's circulation. A drug faces its biggest hurdles during absorption. Medicines taken by mouth are shuttled via a special blood vessel leading from the digestive tract to the liver, where a large amount may be destroyed by metabolic enzymes in the so-called "first-pass effect." Other routes of drug administration bypass the liver, entering the bloodstream directly or via the skin or lungs.

> *Human skin is like a tightly woven fabric, seemingly impervious but porous at the microscopic level. Through its millions of tiny openings, the body oozes sweat and absorbs some substances applied to the skin.*

For a topical agent to be effective obviously it must first be absorbed. The drug must enter in adequate concentration to its proposed site of action to produce the desired response of the skin. This skin is involved in dynamic exchange between the internal and external environments through respiration, absorption, and elimination. It is highly permeable even though it has the ability to maintain its important bacteria-inhibiting barrier with the environment. Individuals vary in the amount of medication they absorb through the skin.

In transdermal medicine substances are applied to the skin's surface and then diffuse out of its vehicle into the stratum corneum (outermost layer of the epidermis). In the stratum corneum (outermost layer of the epidermis) they build a reservoir and defuse through the stratum spinosum, (fourth and thickest layer of the epidermis). At this point, they can be metabolized and bind to receptors thus exerting their effects. Finally, whatever healing or medical substance is applied is delivered into subcutaneous fat, the circulatory system and achieves systemic absorption.

When using transdermal medicines one has to be aware that:

Applying more of a substance increases the amount absorbed. Penetration will stop generally when the skin is saturated. Absorption into the bloodstream is also increased if the concentration of a substance is higher and if more body is covered. Obviously the skin of infants is more prone to absorption than those of adults. Occluded (skin that has been covered) or well-hydrated skin is easier to penetrate than nonoccluded or dry skin.

There are many things that affect skin absorption. Absorption occurs by distribution around and through the cells that make up the skin. Some absorption takes place along hair follicles or through sweat ducts. Skin thickness and barrier accessibility are different in various areas so absorption rates will vary in different parts of the body. For example, hydrocortisone (a synthetic preparation used in the treatment of inflammations, allergies, and itching) is absorbed through the skin 6 times better on the forehead than on the arm, and 44 times better on the scrotum. For this reason, many men can apply iodine to the scrotum, which gets absorbed more intensely than with oral administration. The iodine will rush to the thyroid and back down again to stimulate testosterone, heal the prostate, and in general stimulate desire and bring power to the penis.

Physical condition of the skin at the point of external application is significant. The skin of an infant or child is more permeable than that of adults. The skin over the organs in decreasing order of permeability is genitals, head and neck, trunk, arm and leg. Skin abrasion allows a locally applied substance to come directly in contact with subcutaneous tissue and blood vessels. Absorption is at a much higher rate than in healthy skin. Inflammation leaves the skin leaky and allows larger molecules to be absorbed.

CONCLUSION

In this section you have been provided with reasons why iodine is essential to human health, recommended dosages of iodine, different iodine preparations, and the option and benefits of using iodine transdermally. In the next chapter you will be presented with the negative consequences to your health from the threats of radioactive iodine.

8. How Safe Is Radioactive Iodine-129 and Iodine-131?

We have all been led to believe that radioactive iodine is no longer a threat from Fukushima because it has such a short half-life. However just another proof of a vast cover-up and diminishing of concern over the threat from Fukushima comes from Iodine-129 (I-129), which has a long half-life of 15.7 million years. Thanks to that, the Pacific coast will never be the same. It will take about 16 million years for the contamination from the nuclear accident to dissipate. Radiation apologists diminish the dangers of radioactive iodine because they focus only on Iodine-131 (I-131), which has a short half-life of eight days.

In the 1990s, many studies reported an increase in thyroid cancer in children due to the release of I-131 during the Chernobyl accident in 1986 (Prisyazhniuk et al., 1991; Kazakov et al., 1992). While a vast array of radioactive isotopes were released into the environment during the Fukushima meltdown, I-129 is a particularly concerning material, due to its incredibly long half-life.

The release of I-129 into the environment means that food that comes from the North American western coast will likely be contaminated with radiation for innumerable generations to come. Radiation in the oceans will inevitably enter our water supply and consequently our food supply as well.

According to the Agency for Toxic Substances and Disease Registry (ATSDR), iodine from the ocean enters the air as sea spray or iodine gas. Once in the air iodine can then combine with water particles and enter surface water and soil once the particles fall to ground. Iodine can remain in the soil for extremely long periods of time because it can combine with organic material easily. Plants and vegetation that grow in this soil also have the potential to absorb the iodine.

Dr. Michael Friedman, a leading thyroid and parathyroid expert and surgeon, says, "Women are particularly at risk due to environmental agents depleting iodine reserves and other agents exposing them to radioactive I-131. After the thyroid gland, the distal portions of the human mammary glands are the heaviest users/concentrators of iodine in tissue. Iodine is readily incorporated into the tissues surrounding the mammary nipples and is essential for the maintenance of healthy functioning breast tissue. The radioactive decay of I-131 in breast tissue may be a significant factor in the initiation and progression of both breast cancer and some types of breast nodules."

Radioactive iodine is one of the most harmful radionuclides (an atom with an excess of nuclear energy) because it has the highest activity among radionuclides immediately after an accident, and it causes thyroid cancer in children.

IODINE-129—A GROWING RADIOLOGICAL RISK

Iodine-131 and Iodine-129 travel together, so the presence of the easily detectable short-lived isotope signals the presence of the longer-lived one. "If you have a recent event like Fukushima, you are going to have both present. The Iodine-131 is going to decay away pretty quickly over the course of weeks, but the Iodine-129 is there forever, essentially." Joshua Landis, a research associate in the Department of Earth Science at Dartmouth explains, "Once the Iodine-131 decays, you lose your ability to track the migration of either isotope."

One of the many problems with the official government maps and press releases is that they do not mention radioactive I-129. Not only is this long lived radioactive I-129 dangerous to thyroids, just like it's short lived cousin, it also gets poured out of melting down reactors at a rate that is about 31 times that of the short lived radioactive cousin, I-131. The nuclear industry propaganda machine likes to focus only on the short-lived iodine and ignore the long-lived one, which has serious implications for the future of the human race.

Amazing facts when you consider that 31.6 times as much I-129 than I-131was released in the early days of the Fukushima catastrophe and that was felt as far away as New York, where I -131gas exceeded 3,400 Bq/m^3.

Iodine-129, although a result of nuclear fission in reactors, also occurs to a small extent in the upper atmosphere due to the interaction of high-energy particles with naturally-occurring xenon. "This is very amazing to me, having been working in the radioactive xenon monitoring field for about 17 years now. This was astounding to me . . . You can see background levels around 0.1 mBq/m3 . . . Note the peak concentration we saw was in the range of 45,000 mBq/m3—so that is 450,000 times our background level. For me that's astounding. We never have ever seen anything even close to that. So the concentrations went up and up and up every day, and so it was quite amazing to see this 7,000 kilometers away from the event. I only show some of the data here, but it actually persisted for weeks at very measurable levels, and filled the entire northern hemisphere and mixed into the southern hemisphere," reports one of the researchers on ENE news.

Formation of Radioactive Xenon

Iodine-129 decays into radioactive Xenon-129 sometime during its 16 million years. It is important to realize that radioactive iodine does not disappear. It transmutes as it decays into other radioactive elements, such as radioactive Xenon gas, which can be inhaled easily and which causes lung cancer. Once inhaled, Xenon gas decays into solid radioactive Cesium, which is also cancer causing but in different ways. Then radioactive cesium decays over the next 300 years into other more dangerous, radioactive elements, finally ending with the toxic heavy metal lead, which is extremely toxic and deadly even in small amounts.

Some types of radioactive Xenon is produced from nuclear fission. Other isotopes of Xenon are produced by beta decay, meaning heightened world levels of Xenon are a symptom of numerous other types of radioactive particles decaying in the broad environment.

Effects on the Body

According to the Environmental Protection Agency when I-129 or I-131 is ingested, some of it concentrates in the thyroid gland. The rest passes from the body in urine. Airborne I-129 and I-131 can be inhaled. In the lung, radioactive iodine is absorbed, passes into the blood stream, and collects in the thyroid.

In the body, iodine has a biological half-life of about 100 days for the body as a whole. It has different biological half-lives for various organs: thyroid—100 days, bone—14 days, and kidney, spleen, and reproductive organs—7 days.

Iodine-129 and Iodine-131 experience beta decay, which means they emit beta particles when decaying from unstable to stable form. Beta particles are moderately energetic. Gamma rays are also emitted and are highly energetic, which means that they can be detected outside the body. Beta particles easily pass through soft tissue and cause damage to DNA by shattering DNA strands and knocking out chunks of gene sequences.

Effects on the Environment

"Due to its long half-life and continued release from ongoing nuclear energy production, Iodine-129 is perpetually accumulating in the environment and poses a growing radiological risk," the authors of a study at Dartmouth point out. It is important to note that I-129 was already present before the Fukushima Daiichi accident owing to atmospheric nuclear testing held in the 1950s and 1960s, and later, discharged from spent-nuclear-fuel reprocessing plants.

Iodine-129 has leaked into groundwater at nuclear weapons production locations, including the Hanford Site in Washington State. Meanwhile, France and England—which produce large proportions of their electricity via nuclear power—are reprocessing spent fuel and disposing of vast quantities of Iodine-129 simply by dumping it in the ocean.

Ocean disposal of Iodine-129 appears to have resulted in massive increases of radionuclide concentrations. Currents carry the British and French Iodine-129 northward, and a 2003 Danish study found concentrations in the Kattegat strait between Denmark and Sweden increased six fold between 1992 and 2000. Concentrations of Iodine-129 in some Arctic waters are 4,000 times their pre-nuclear era levels.

The Fukushima Daiichi nuclear power plant released an enormous amount of liquid waste of Iodine-129 and other fission isotopes directly into the Pacific Ocean that were and continue to be dispersed eastwards.

Most of the radiation resulting from Fukushima was washed out to sea and it is quickly destroying the Pacific Ocean and much of the life in it. We have no idea how much of the radiation is escaping into the atmosphere, but we do know that during the first few weeks of the nuclear accident, because of the explosions, huge amounts of radiation were released into the atmosphere, and it circled around the globe especially in the northern hemisphere.

TREATMENT/PREVENTION OF POISONING FROM RADIOACTIVE IODINE

It is important to remember that iodine supplementation diminishes the dangers of ionized radiation. Dr. Brownstein writes, "If there is enough inorganic, non-radioactive iodine in our bodies, the radioactive fallout has nowhere to bind in our bodies. It will pass through us, leaving our bodies unharmed. It is important to ensure that we have adequate iodine levels before fallout hits."

Dangers When Used for Cancer Treatments

Cancer rates go up with increasing levels of radiation and heavy metal contamination. Most people, including doctors, ignore the dangers of using radiation in medicine. The medical establishment is incapable of responding to the nuclear threat and the spreading contamination from Japan because it is an institution that uses dangerous levels of radiation to diagnosis and treat cancer and other diseases.

When it comes to using radiation to treat cancer they administer near to lethal dosages and they wonder why so many people die. The average lifetime dose of diagnostic radiation has increased sevenfold since 1980 with doctors and dentists having no real idea of the risks they are taking with their patients' lives.

Thyroid Cancer

There was a large increase in the proportion of thyroid cancer patients receiving radioactive iodine between 1990 and 2008 even though radioactive iodine is a cause of thyroid cancer. Between 1990 and 2008, the percentage of patients treated with radioactive iodine climbed from 40 to 56 percent. According to the *Journal of the American Medical Association*, there are more than 40,000 new cases of thyroid cancer every year in the U.S.—a number that has been climbing steadily.

Overtreatment of thyroid cancer with radioactive iodine is rampant even though there is substantial uncertainty about the indications for its use and safety for the treatment of thyroid cancer. Radioactive iodine absorbed by the thyroid can injure the gland. According to a new study published in *Cancer*, researchers are fingering doctors who are treating patients with early-stage, low-risk thyroid cancer using radioactive iodine, which does not increase their chances of surviving but does put them at risk for a secondary cancer. "Our study shows that these low-risk patients do not need radioactive iodine," Dr. Ian Ganly, one of the study's authors from Memorial Sloan-Kettering Cancer Center in New York, told Reuters Health. "Therefore there is no need to expose these patients to any risk from (radioactive iodine) treatment," he said.

The American Thyroid Association endorses the use of radioactive iodine even though it also causes cancer of the salivary gland—where radioactive iodine may accumulate—as well as leukemia. Dr. Ganly said the risk of leukemia increases because radioactive iodine circulates in the blood, thus exposing bone marrow to its tissue-killing effects.

*Because iodine deficiency results in increased iodine trapping
by the thyroid, iodine deficient individuals of all ages are
more susceptible to radiation-induced thyroid cancer.*

The downsides of radioactive iodine are clear: the therapy saps patients' energy and ups their risk of developing new cancers down the road, and it costs thousands of dollars. "There are a lot of patients who are receiving radioactive iodine for what is considered low-risk tumors," said Dr. David J. Sher, a cancer expert at Rush University Medical Center in Chicago. "These patients generally have a superb prognosis without radioactive iodine."

On orthodox medical sites we will read, *The Cause of Thyroid Cancer is Unknown.* Nobody wants to step out and just say that iodine deficiency can cause thyroid cancer. Some sites do say that certain risk factors for thyroid cancer include:

- A history of thyroid disease (iodine deficiency)

- An inherited abnormal gene or a bowel condition called FAP (Familial Adenomatous Polyposis)

- Exposure to radiation, especially in childhood

- Goiter (iodine deficiency)

- Iodine deficiency

People who have low iodine levels are more likely to get thyroid cancer than those who do not. "Over a third of children in Japan's Fukushima region could be prone to cancer if medics don't apply more effort in treating their unusually overgrown thyroid glands." A report shows that nearly 36 percent of children in the nuclear-disaster-affected Fukushima Prefecture have abnormal thyroid growths. After examining more than 38,000 children from the area, medics found that more than 13,000 have cysts or nodules as large as 5 millimeters on their thyroids, the Sixth Report of Fukushima Prefecture Health Management Survey states.

We also know, though the government is not telling anyone, that the initial high levels of radioactive iodine hit both coasts of American and was reported further on in Europe as well during the initial month of the disaster. Pediatrician Helen Caldecott said, "The data should be made available. And they should be consulting with international experts ASAP. And the lesions on the ultrasounds should all be biopsied, and they're not being biopsied. And if they're not being biopsied, then that's ultimately medical irresponsibility. Because if some of these children have cancer and they're not treated, they're going to die."

Radiation Poisoning May Lead To Congenital Hypothyroidism. The World Health Organization warns that young people are particularly prone to radiation poisoning in the thyroid gland. Infants face the direst consequences, as their cells divide at a higher rate. It is believed that some children were exposed to "lifetime" doses of radiation to their thyroid glands, says a report by Japan's Institute of Radiological Sciences.

A new study from the Radiation and Public Health Project found that babies born in the western United States as well as other Pacific countries shortly after the Fukushima nuclear disaster in Japan in March 2011 might be at greater risk for congenital hypothyroidism. According to the U.S. National Library of Medicine, "If untreated, congenital hypothyroidism can lead to intellectual disability and abnormal growth."

Why Doctors Don't Say More About Radiation Dangers

Doctors are among the primary users of nuclear radiation, using it for all kinds of dangerous tests. A single CT scan of the chest is equal to about 350 standard chest X-rays. They are using radiation, a cause of cancer, to try to treat cancer and that usually does not turn out too well. Because they are not honest with themselves they cannot be honest with their patients, who should be told that many of the tests they are being given by doctors expose them to more dangerous radiation.

When was the last time you remember your doctor telling you to drink lots of iodine, or take magnesium or sodium bicarbonate, and start off each day drinking a glass of ultra-pure edible clay or even sulfur to reduce the risk that our exposure to increasing levels of radiation do not lead to cancer. Edible clay is one of the most basic detoxification substances. It helps make sure absorbed radioactive particles pass through, instead of into us.

CONCLUSION

Like global warming and vaccines, there is no real discussion, no real science being sported in the news, so the public is left completely in the dark about radiation exposures. The people with the real power in this world insist that we will always see and define the situation as safe, no need to worry or do anything. However, as you have read in this chapter there are dangers that are of concern when exposed to radiation.

The next section Part 3 of the book deals with maintaining healthy organs, beginning with your thyroid gland, and treatments for conditions. Chapter 9 outlines how critical iodine is in order for the thyroid gland to function properly.

PART THREE
Conditions and Treatments

9. Iodine and the Thyroid Gland

The thyroid gland is a butterfly-shaped endocrine gland that is normally located in the lower front of the neck, see Figure 9.1. The thyroid's job is to make thyroid hormone, which is secreted into the blood and then carried to every tissue in the body. Thyroid hormone is essential to help each cell in each tissue and organ to work right. For example, thyroid hormone helps the body use energy, stay warm, and keep the brain, heart, muscles, and other organs working as they should.

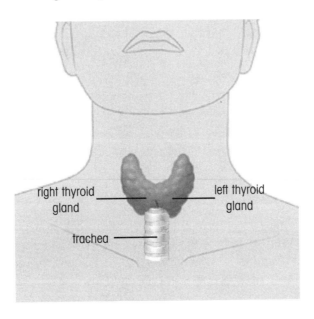

Figure 9.1. Thyroid Gland

While the thyroid gland contains the body's highest concentration of iodine, the salivary glands, brain, cerebrospinal fluid, gastric mucosa, breasts, ovaries, and a part of the eye also concentrate iodine. In the brain, iodine is found in the choroid plexus, the area on the ventricles of the brain where cerebrospinal fluid (CSF) is produced, and in the substantia nigra, an area associated with Parkinson's disease.

Every 17 minutes, every drop of blood in our body flushes through our thyroid, and if our thyroid has an adequate supply of iodine, blood-borne bacteria and viruses are killed off as the blood passes through the thyroid.

Iodine is critical to the function of the thyroid. In fact, it is iodine and the amino acid L-tyrosine that creates thyroid hormone. As fluoride has a lower molecular weight than iodine, it can disrupt the function of thyroid hormone thus contributing to hypothyroid conditions. Thus, fluoride lowers metabolism, which decreases the efficiency of approximately 3,000 enzymes.

Iodine made its leap into medical history when a Swiss physician, Jean François Condet announced that iodine could reduce goiters (enlarged thyroids). At this moment, modern medical science was born because for the first time we have a specific disorder that is relieved by a specific treatment. It is most ironic to note that the very first step of allopathic medicine was into nutritional not chemical medicine with iodine being a common mineral from the sea.

The required daily amount (RDA) of iodine is just enough to keep our thyroids from expanding, like the RDA of vitamin C today, which is just enough to keep us free of scurvy but not enough to prevent pre-scurvy syndromes or Cardiovascular Disease.

THYROID HORMONES

The thyroid gland, located in the base of the neck in a typical body, is involved in secreting important hormones T4 (thyroxine) and T3 (triiodothyronine). T3 contains 3 iodine atoms and is created from the breakdown of T4. The breakdown of T4 is encouraged by the thyroid stimulating hormone.

T4 is synthesized from residues of the amino acid tyrosine, found in thyroglobulin (a protein created in the thyroid). It contains four iodine atoms. T4 allows the body to control the more active T3 better. If there is too much of the thyroid hormones in the bloodstream, the hypothalamus will signal the pituitary gland (via TRH) to produce TSH for the thyroid to release more T3 and T4. Once there is enough of these hormones the hypothalamus will be signaled to stop the release of TRH and the cascade of actions to increase T3 and T4.

Inorganic non-radioactive iodine/iodide is an essential nutrient, not a drug. Therefore, the body has the metabolic mechanism for using inorganic iodine beneficially, effectively, and safely. Iodine is as safe as magnesium chloride with a record of accomplishment of 180 years of use in medicine.

Iodine is needed in microgram amounts for the thyroid, mg amounts for breast and other tissues, and can be used therapeutically in gram amounts.

—Dr. David Miller, Iodine for Health

Published data confirms its safety even when used in pulmonary patients in amounts four orders of magnitude greater than the U.S. RDA. When patients take between 12.5 to 50 mg of iodine per day, it seems that the body becomes increasingly more responsive to thyroid hormones. Optimal intake of iodine in amounts two orders of magnitude greater than iodine levels needed for goiter control may be required for iodization of hormone receptors.

Iodine helps us utilize our proteins properly. In all likelihood an iodine deficient person will remain protein deficient.

—Dr. Brice Vickery, Chiropractor

Thyroxin and Triiodothyronine stimulates and maintains normal heart rate, blood pressure and body temperature. "Despite the general medical dependence upon special hormone tests, such as TSH, temperature appears to be much more accurate for assessing thyroid function. During the past decade, I have noticed that 90 percent of individuals have a temperature BELOW normal. The oral temperature before getting out of bed in the morning should be 97.6 degrees Fahrenheit or higher. Mid-afternoon the temperature should be 98.6. Temperature is the simplest measure of basal metabolic rate, the key function of the thyroid gland," said Dr. Norman Shealy.

Physiological Effects

Thyroid hormones have two major physiological effects. They increase protein synthesis in virtually every body tissue and increase oxygen consumption dependent upon Na^+-K^+ ATPase (Na pump). The thyroid gland needs iodine to synthesize thyroxine (T4) and triiodothyronine (T3), hormones that regulate metabolism and steer growth and development. Thyroid hormones are essential for life as they regulate key biochemical reactions, especially protein synthesis and enzymatic activities, in target organs, such as the developing brain, muscle, heart, pituitary, and kidney; thus iodine is critically important to the developing fetus.

The thyroid hormones are synthesized in the follicular cells of the thyroid. The first step to hormone synthesis is the import of iodide into the follicular cells. Thyroid hormone regulates mitochondrial protein synthesis through the stimulation of synthesis of mitochondrial protein synthesis modulators, and that the tissue specific modulators (stimulatory in liver and inhibitory in kidney) can be produced by the hormone. Whole body iodine sufficiency is a critical means to counter the side effects of thyroid hormone medications (such as Synthroid). Long-term use of these drugs is associated with depletion of thyroid and tissue iodine levels, as well as increased rates of cancer. All thyroid patients should be on iodine therapy.

MEDICINAL AND BIOLOGIC EFFECTS OF IODINE

Iodine is a powerful primary nutrient with broad medicinal effects and 100 years ago it was used universally by most doctors. From 1900 to the 1960s almost every single U.S. physician used Lugol (iodine) supplements in his or her practice for both hypo and hyperthyroid, as well as many, many other conditions, all with excellent results. In fact, iodine was considered a panacea for all human ills. The Nobel laureate Dr. Albert Szent Györgi (1893–1986), the physician who discovered vitamin C, writes: "When I was a medical student, iodine in the form of KI (potassium iodide) was the universal medicine. Nobody knew what it did, but it did something and did something good." Today we know what iodine does and how much it can help people, but modern allopathic medicine is asleep at the switch letting people suffer and die for its lacking.

"Breast, ovarian, and skin cysts—In addition to fixing almost all cases of breast cysts, iodine also has a remarkable healing effect on ovarian cysts," says Dr. Robert Rowen. Though few know it, swollen ovaries is a condition analogous to goiter, when the thyroid swells in response to iodine deficiency. Goiters often also result in a hormonal imbalance leading to hypothyroidism. In the case of Polycystic Ovary Syndrome (PCOS) the starvation of the ovaries causes them to become cystic, swollen, and eventually unable to regulate the synthesis of their hormones leading to imbalances and infertility.

Breast tissue has an affinity for iodine. Iodine deficiency causes fibrocystic breast disease with nodules, cyst enlargement, pain, and scar tissue.

Russian studies, when investigating Fibrocystic breast disease also discovered that the greater the iodine deficiency the greater the number of cysts in the ovaries. Since 1928, the iodine concentration in the ovary has been known to be higher than in every other organ except the thyroid. Dr. Browstein has found in his research with high doses of iodine that cysts on the ovaries became smaller and began to disappear. He also found that libido in women and men increased.

Iodine has many non-endocrine biologic effects, including the role it plays in the physiology of the inflammatory response. Iodides increase the movement of granulocytes into areas of inflammation and improve the phagocytosis of bacteria by granulocytes and the ability of granulocytes to kill bacteria.

Dr. Robert Rowen informs that iodine reduces the activity of lipoprotein(a). When elevated, this protein can lead to excessive blood clotting and vascular disease. Iodine has been used successfully in headaches, keloid formation, parotid duct stones, and Dupuytren's and Peyronie's contractures. Doses up to six times the RDA have been used safely for months to combat the excessive mucous in chronic lung diseases. He also states that iodine is found in large amounts in the brain (including the parts of the brain associated with Parkinson's disease) and the ciliary body of the eye, a possible factor in glaucoma.

"One 1860 French physician mistakenly gave a tincture of iodine when he meant to give digitalis to a woman with Grave's Disease. She recovered within 3 weeks. When he discovered his mistake, he switched to digitalis, and her symptoms came back. He switched back to the iodine and achieved a remission," reported Dr. Rowen.

"We placed an 83-year-old woman on orthoiodo-supplementation [daily amount of iodine required for whole body sufficiency] for 6 months at 50 mgs of elemental iodine daily. She experienced a tremendous increase in energy, endurance, well-being, and memory. At 6 months all her skin peeled off and was replaced by new, younger-looking skin. She was flabbergasted and amazed at her new appearance. In our experience older women (especially over 65) noticed a major difference both physically and mentally," wrote Dr. Guy Abraham, an endocrinologist who today is providing the backbone of the movement back toward the use of iodine as an essential safe and effective medicine.

Drs. Abraham, Flechas, and Brownstein tested more than 4,000 patients taking iodine in daily doses ranging from 12.5 to 50 mg, and in those with diabetes, up to 100 mg a day. These investigators found that "iodine does indeed reverse fibrocystic disease; their diabetic patients require less insulin; hypothyroid patients, less thyroid medication; symptoms of fibromyalgia resolve, and patients with migraine headaches stop having them." We can expect even better results when iodine is combined with magnesium chloride.

Iodine is utilized by every hormone receptor in the body. The absence of iodine causes a hormonal dysfunction that can be seen with practically every hormone inside the body.

—Dr. Jorge Flechas

Why did Dr. Flechas see such dramatic results with his diabetic patients? The most obvious answer is that iodine is a trace mineral used to synthesize hormones and is a mineral that is very important to how hormones function at the hormone receptor sites.

Iodine's ability to revive hormonal sensitivity seems to significantly improve insulin sensitivity. Dr. Flechas said, "It was while treating a large 320-pound woman with insulin dependent diabetes that we learned a valuable lesson regarding the role of iodine in hormone receptor function. This woman had come in via the emergency room with a very high random blood sugar of 1,380 mg/dl. She was then started on insulin during her hospitalization and was instructed on the use of a home glucometer. She was to use her glucometer two times per day. Two weeks later on her return office visit for a checkup of her insulin dependent diabetes she was informed that during her hospital physical examination she was noted to have FBD [fibrocystic breast disease]. She was recommended to start on 50 mg of iodine (4 tablets) at that time. One week later she called us requesting to lower the level of insulin due to having problems with hypoglycemia. She was told to continue to drop her insulin levels as long as she was experiencing hypoglycemia and to monitor her blood sugars carefully with her glucometer. Four weeks later during an office visit her glucometer was downloaded to my office computer, which showed her to have an average random blood sugar of 98. I praised the patient for her diligent efforts to control her diet and her good work at keeping her sugars under control with the insulin. She then informed me that she had come off her insulin three weeks earlier and had not been taking any medications to lower her blood sugar. When asked what she felt the big change was, she felt that her diabetes was under better control due to the use of iodine."

Increased metabolic rate increases the need for iodine. If a person is not getting enough iodine and are on thyroid meds they will become more deficient.

—Dr. Jorge Flechas

Dr. Fletchas reported that 2 years later and 70 pounds lighter this above patient continues to have excellent glucose control on iodine, 50 mg per day. "We since have done a study of twelve diabetics and in six cases we were able to wean all of these patients off of medications for their diabetes. The range of daily iodine intake was from 50 mg to 100 mg per day. All diabetic patients were able to lower the total amount of medications necessary to control their diabetes."

Iodine is my drug of choice. I use it for everything. I raised my kids and now my grandkids on iodine. My son was due to have his tonsils removed and I decided to paint his tonsils and he has never had any more problems with his throat. I took a spray bottle and poured some iodine into the bottle and sprayed his tonsils. As you may know iodine dries quickly, so he didn't really swallow any. It worked within 24 hours after spraying the throat.

According to Dr. John Myer iodine has a marked effect on muscle contraction directly. It relieves cramps of the leg muscles known as "charley horses". It also relieves pain in the pericardium (membrane enclosing the heart), and it has a remarkable effect on muscle energy and contraction of all muscles of the body. Dr. Myer also asserts that iodine plays a decisive and critical role in the lymph system and in the lymph glands. Swollen sub maxillary glands, known as "waxen kernels" to our parents and grandparents, will soften and regress within minutes after allowing iodized lime to dissolve in the mouth.

I tried Iodoral for 10 days. I began with the full 50 mg and did this for five days. I felt very bad the whole time, had skin eruptions and a light reddish rash on my face, depressed, considerable sneezing, and finally ended up with a sinus headache that was close to a migraine. And this was after cutting back to 25 mg/day. When I stopped, I immediately felt better.

When one combines the intake of iodine with other minerals (iodine in combination with selenium increased the activities of type 1 deiodinase (D1) and glutathione peroxidase (GSHPx) one can expect strong and positive changes in cell physiology.

Iodine and/or selenium deficiency may modify the distribution and the homeostasis of other minerals.

Dr. Daniel H. Duffy employs some unkind but warranted words while questioning the use of iodine, "Isn't it odd that the government dispenses iodine to protect against radioactive iodine resulting from a nuclear disaster when the medical quacks are dumping the same type of radioactive iodine into patients with thyroid problems in a stupid attempt to "cure" thyroid "disease" caused by a lack of elemental iodine in its natural state found in nature? Nature's iodine protects our thyroid glands from taking up biologically destructive, radioactive iodine, yet the medical quacks use similar radioactive iodine to destroy our thyroid glands? Why did doctors quit using Lugol's solution, the sure cure for thyroid disease? Why did the medical quacks bring in anti-thyroid drugs and goitrogens to kill the thyroid gland when iodine was being used so successfully for so long?"

ORTHOIODOSUPPLEMENTATION

Orthoiodosupplementation employs elemental supplements until the thyroid gland and all other iodine-sensitive sites in the body have reached iodine sufficiency. In reality there is no reason to fear iodine if approached with reason and a slight bit of caution, for it will stimulate a detoxification process of heavy metals especially of halogens. All doctors used iodine 100 years ago and the best ones are still using it today.

Orthoiodosupplementation should be part of a complete nutritional program, emphasizing magnesium instead of calcium.

—Dr. Guy Abraham

Is Taking Iodine Good or Bad for Hashimoto's Disease?

There has been quite a bit of controversy over whether Hashimoto's patients should take supplemental iodine. Many of the doctors quoted in this book advocate mega doses of iodine, up to a hundred times the recommended daily dose or more. Most people have no problem with taking high dosages of iodine, but there are doctors who believe that extremely high levels of iodine can actually cause both hyperthyroidism and hypothyroidism. This might be true with the accent on the word extreme, which would include not just dosages but length of time at high dosages.

Mainstream physicians argue against Hashimoto's patients taking iodine supplements because they believe that if you have Hashimoto's your system already has too much iodine and that more will only make your condition worse. With doctors like Brownstein finding 97 percent of patients being iodine deficient, one has to wonder where this excess iodine is coming from.

It is more likely that iodine substitutes like fluoride, chlorine, and bromide are causing the problem. Heavy exposure to these three chemicals mean that we aren't getting as much iodine as we think we are because they replace iodine without providing any of the positive and necessary effects of iodine. These common chemicals cause us to be low in iodine.

Our bodies are incredibly efficient at absorbing and storing iodine. Unfortunately, our thyroids cannot tell the difference between iodine and other substances with very similar chemical structures. Iodine is part of the halogen family, which also includes fluorine, chlorine, and bromine. They all fall into the same column of the periodic table meaning they have very similar properties. Fluorine, chlorine, and bromine are similar enough to iodine that your thyroid will suck them up and store them in place of iodine, effectively "displacing" iodine, especially when we are deficient in iodine making the thyroid desperate for anything that even looks like iodine.

These fake iodine replacements cannot be used to make thyroid hormones. If fluorine, chlorine, and bromine are displacing iodine, your thyroid will not have enough iodine to produce thyroid hormones, which can lead to hypothyroidism and Hashimoto's. The higher the concentration of these chemicals that you have in your body, and the lower your iodine levels are, the more likely it is that your thyroid levels will be low and you will experience Hashimoto's symptoms, such as fatigue, brain fog, weight gain, hair loss, and more. Unfortunately, these three chemicals are now frequently added to our water, foods, and household products creating medical problems of unmeasurable and unfathomable levels.

Do Not Use Radioactive Iodine
to Treat Thyroid Cancer

Cancer rates go up with increasing levels of radiation and heavy metal contamination. Most people, including doctors, ignore the dangers of using radiation in medicine. The medical establishment is an institution that uses dangerous levels of radiation to diagnose and treat cancer and other diseases. The average lifetime dose of diagnostic radiation has increased sevenfold since 1980 with doctors and dentists having no real idea of the risks they are taking with their patients' lives.

There was a large increase in the proportion of thyroid cancer patients receiving radioactive iodine between 1990 and 2008 even though radioactive iodine is a cause of thyroid cancer. Between 1990 and 2008, the percentage of patients treated with radioactive iodine climbed from 40 to 56 percent. According to the *Journal of the American Medical Association*, there are more than 40,000 new cases of thyroid cancer every year in the U.S.—a number that has been climbing steadily.

Overtreatment of thyroid cancer with radioactive iodine is rampant, even though there is substantial uncertainty about the indications for its use and safety for the treatment of thyroid cancer. Radioactive iodine absorbed by the thyroid can injure the gland. According to a new study published in *Cancer*, researchers are fingering doctors who are treating patients with early-stage, low-risk thyroid cancer using radioactive iodine, which does not increase their chances of surviving but does put them at risk for a secondary cancer. "Our study shows that these low-risk patients do not need radioactive iodine," Dr. Ian Ganly, one of the study's authors from Memorial Sloan-Kettering Cancer Center in New York, told Reuters Health. "Therefore there is no need to expose these patients to any risk from (radioactive iodine) treatment," he said.

Iodine, Thyroid, And Low Body Temperature

Who will benefit from taking iodine? Actually, the answer is just about everyone will benefit from more iodine. Did you know that over 30 percent of the U.S. has thyroid problems and that is probably a huge underestimate considering how iodine deficient the population is in the United States and around the world.

The American Thyroid Association endorses the use of radioactive iodine even though it also causes cancer of the salivary gland—where radioactive iodine may accumulate—as well as leukemia. Dr. Ganly said the risk of leukemia increases because radioactive iodine circulates in the blood, thus exposing bone marrow to its tissue-killing effects.

Because iodine deficiency results in increased iodine trapping by the thyroid, iodine deficient individuals of all ages are more susceptible to radiation-induced thyroid cancer.

The downsides of radioactive iodine are clear: The therapy saps patients' energy and ups their risk of developing new cancers down the road, and it costs thousands of dollars. "There are a lot of patients who are receiving radioactive iodine for what is considered low-risk tumors," said Dr. David J. Sher, a cancer expert at Rush University Medical Center in Chicago. "These patients generally have a superb prognosis without radioactive iodine."

On orthodox medical sites we will read, "The Cause of Thyroid Cancer is Unknown." Nobody wants to step out and just say that iodine deficiency can cause thyroid cancer. Some sites do say that certain risk factors for thyroid cancer include:

• A history of thyroid disease (iodine deficiency)

• Exposure to radiation, especially in childhood

• An inherited abnormal gene or a bowel condition called FAP

• Iodine Deficiency

• Goiter (iodine deficiency)

People who have low iodine levels are more likely to get thyroid cancer than those who do not.

The best method to diagnose the condition of your thyroid is not a blood test but is to take your temperature. Just take your oral temperature a few times daily. If your temperature is not 98.6, but instead runs lower, then the latest thyroid research says that your thyroid needs treatment. Unfortunately, doctors often overlook low body temperature as a serious sign of disease.

*Iodine is the agent, which arouses (kindles) and keeps going the flame
of life. With the aid of our thyroid, in which the iodine is manifesting,
it can either damp this flame or kindle it to a dissolute fire.*

—Scholz 1990

Iodine is the primary treatment for thyroid conditions. It is as the coal shoveled into the engines of a might ship. Iodine lights the fire, not only of the thyroid, but also through the function of thyroid hormones, the fires of every cell in the body.

When the body does not have enough energy and heat to function properly, many things begin to go wrong. For example, if the brain has too little energy, thought processes, such as memory and focus, become impaired. The body needs energy to keep itself warm—a low body temperature, therefore, usually accompanies low metabolic energy.

The primary symptoms of under-active thyroid functions include:

- Bipolar disease ($^2/_3$ of all bipolar patients become normal with correction to normal thyroid activity)
- Cold hands and feet (low body temperature)
- Constipation
- Dry skin
- Fatigue
- Fluid retention, depression
- Fuzzy thinking
- Low blood pressure
- Slow reflexes
- Underweight or overweight

When using high-dose iodine supplements watch out for signs of over-active thyroid functions. These include:

- Anxiety
- Bulging eye and vision disturbances
- Diarrhea
- High blood pressure
- High pulse rate
- Insomnia
- Rapid weight loss
- Sensitivity

Core Body Temperature

Temperature is an indicator of the amount of heat contained in a system, and our temperature is an extension of basic body metabolism. Heat is a form of energy and every reaction in a human body occurs at a certain energy or temperature level thus tracking with cell voltage and pH and oxygen levels, see Table 9.1 on page 110.

The core body temperature of a human body is an important factor, which is always why it should be considered while evaluating the health condition in a checkup. Normal core temperatures are at the exact temperature at which all the functions of the human body can operate with optimal efficiency. The same can be said about pH because all physiological processes are pH sensitive. The same can be said about oxygen levels and thus the quality of our breathing, something we do correctly or not 24/7.

Normally the rectal temperature or vaginal temperature is considered as the core temperature. The ideal core temperature is considered to be around 98.6° Fahrenheit (F) or 37° Celsius (C). However, this temperature is an average body temperature because the overall normal temperature varies from a minimum of 97.7° F (36.5° C) to a maximum of almost 99.5° F (37.5° C). Any temperature above or below this range is abnormal. Actually, the best time and way of establishing one's basal body temperature is to take it first thing in the morning before getting out of bed.

Dr. David Jernigan says, "Much emphasis in conventional medicine is usually placed upon feverish conditions; however, a low body temperature can be a much more sinister condition. Where a fever can be viewed as an active developmental and corrective process of the healthy body, a low body temperature can never be viewed as a normal or healthy condition, nor is it a mechanism for a learning or developmental process in the body. The colder a body becomes, the slower the electrical oscillatory rate and therefore the thicker, more viscous or syrupy the body fluids become. The more viscous the fluids become the more difficult it is for the body to push the fluids through the body. The lymph fluids that are normally supposed to bathe the outsides of all of your cells become progressively stagnant as it is too thick to move efficiently."

The colder we get the happier viruses, bacteria, and fungi are. Cancer loves cold conditions and dies when things get too hot. The problem with clearing cancer cells, which are always occurring somewhere in the body, even under normal conditions, is that there is no effective immune response when we are too cold. In general, when we are iodine and thyroid deficient it is hard for the body to generate a fever, so chronic infections go undetected and cancer goes forward until we are in a desperate condition.

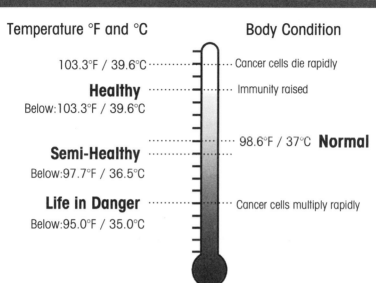

FIGURE 9.1. BODY TEMPERATURE DETERMINES YOUR HEALTH

Temperature °F and °C   Body Condition

103.3°F / 39.6°C ············ Cancer cells die rapidly

Healthy ············ Immunity raised

Below:103.3°F / 39.6°C

············ 98.6°F / 37°C **Normal**

Semi-Healthy ············

Below:97.7°F / 36.5°C

Life in Danger ············ Cancer cells multiply rapidly

Below:95.0°F / 35.0°C

Extreme cold is a dangerous situation that can bring on health emergencies in susceptible people. Cold is a known source of disease and death. Chinese medicine for thousands of years recognized cold as a principle cause of disease. Cold can be either an internal condition due to iodine deficiency and thyroid dysfunction or it can be exposure to cold. Either way it is important to understand and treat cold body conditions.

The easiest, safest, and most effective way of treating most disease, including cancer, is to increase body temperature with infrared therapy and to supplement with plenty of iodine. Both are foundational treatments, which have profound ramifications for thyroid sufferers, patients with adrenal issues, and even for people with restless leg syndrome. Doctors waste a lot of their time and patients' money administering other treatments, which cannot work as long as core body temperature is not raised.

The ideal body temperature for optimal health is 98.6° F. That temperature is the guarantor for good blood circulation and is the mainstay for vitality and strong immune system strength. Low temperatures between 94.1° to 96.8° F is common with most patients with chronic illnesses. It is not too difficult to deduct that a cold person is an ill person.

Cancer tumors grow faster when the body temperature is low. Germany's bestselling author Uwe Karstädt's new book *98.6° F—Ideal Body temperature for Optimal Health* offers a wealth of knowledge and a cut through method of maintaining health or returning to it once we have succumbed to low body temperature and chronic disease. According to the author, low temperature is a plague of the 21st century.

Enzyme Activity

"Coldness in the body is much more than a bothersome and inconvenient symptom. Coldness makes us sick. This coldness, which causes such enormous discomfort in the majority of my patients, is not a trivial matter. Warmth within the body is like the sun for our life here on earth. An indication of vibrant health, strength, and vitality is a body temperature of 98.6° F. We are "hot," full of glowing love when we reproduce; the Grim Reaper, however, takes our life from us with an icy hand. The summer of life is warm and vibrant while winter silences life, burying it under snow and ice," writes Karstädt.

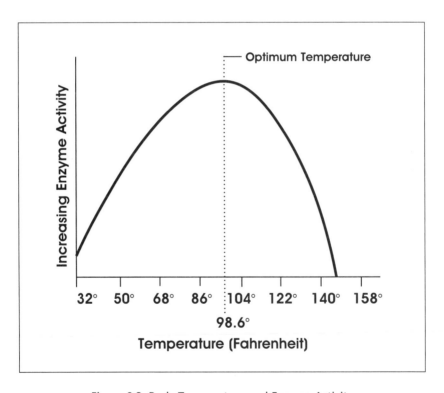

Figure 9.2. Body Temperature and Enzyme Activity

When we look at the fact that lower body temperature decreases enzyme activity (see Table 9.2), we can appreciate how important it is medically speaking to maintain optimal body heat. "Give me fever and I can cure every disease," said Hippocrates 2,500 years ago.

Raising the body temperature is synonymous with an increased immune response. Professor Abo from Japan confirmed a 40 percent improvement in the function of the immune system by raising the body temperature by only 1.8° F.

Besides iodine supplementation a Biomat offers one of the best treatments for cold conditions and is instrumental in treating cancer because of the increased immune response. One can spend a hundred thousand dollars today for sophisticated toxic chemo drugs designed to increase immune system function, or one can purchase a Biomat for between seven hundred and seventeen hundred dollars depending on the size. (http://medicalbiomats.com)

CONCLUSION

As presented in this chapter, iodine deficiency continues to be an important public health issue. Since the body does not produce iodine, iodine supplementation is needed for the production of thyroid hormone and for the well-being of your body.

A sufficient body temperature is more than just a cozy and pleasant feeling. Proper body heat is one of the fundamental pillars of good health. It is also essential to maintain core body temperature for normal functioning of the human body. The important role iodine and selenium play in heart health is made available in the next chapter.

10. Iodine and Selenium for Heart Health

According to *Scientific American*, physicians for decades have grappled with ways to block further tissue damage in patients who suffer heart attacks. They have tried everything from drugs to cell therapy—all with little luck. However, promising research indicates that a bio gel made from seaweed may have the healing powers that have thus far eluded them. Some of the principle healing agents in seaweed are magnesium, iodine, and selenium. Seaweeds with high amounts of iodine have exceptional value in the treatment of the heart, but it is better and safer to use a liquid iodine, magnesium, and selenium at high dosages.

Differences in geographic iodine intake have been shown to be associated with the prevalence of hypothyroidism and hyperthyroidism. Both of these thyroid abnormalities have been shown to negatively affect cardiovascular function. Selenium, an important antioxidant in the thyroid and involved in the metabolism of iodine-containing thyroid hormones, may play an interactive role in the development of these thyroid irregularities, and in turn, cardiovascular disease.

Endemic goiter was common in people and in domestic animals, particularly in the eastern part of Finland away from the sea. Studies in the 1950s revealed that the major dietary difference between eastern and western Finland was iodine. The risk of death from coronary heart disease was 3.5 times higher for people with a goiter in Finland.

THYROID HORMONE DEFICIENCY

"Thyroid hormone is an important regulator of cardiac function and cardiovascular hemodynamics. Triiodothyronine, T3, the physiologically active form of thyroid hormone, binds to nuclear receptor proteins and mediates the expression of several important cardiac genes, inducing transcription of the positively regulated genes, including alpha-myosin heavy chain (MHC) and the sarcoplasmic reticulum calcium ATPase. Negatively regulated genes include beta-MHC and phospholamban, which are down regulated in the presence of normal serum levels of thyroid hormone. T3 mediated effects on the systemic vasculature include relaxation of vascular smooth muscle resulting in decreased arterial resistance and diastolic blood pressure.

In hyperthyroidism, cardiac contractility and cardiac output are enhanced and systemic vascular resistance is decreased, while in hypothyroidism, the opposite is true. Patients with subclinical hypothyroidism manifest many of the same cardiovascular changes, but to a lesser degree than that which occurs in overt hypothyroidism. Cardiac disease states are sometimes associated with the low T3 syndrome. The phenotype of the failing heart resembles that of the hypothyroid heart, both in cardiac physiology and in gene expression. Changes in serum T(3) levels in patients with chronic congestive heart failure are caused by alterations in thyroid hormone metabolism suggesting that patients may benefit from T(3) replacement in this setting."

Iodine-containing thyroid hormones, thyroxine (T4) and triiodothyronine (T3) are important metabolic regulators of cardiovascular activity with the ability to exert action on cardiac myocytes, vascular smooth muscle, and endothelial cells.

—Dr. Stephen. Hoption Cann, Department of Health Care and Epidemiology, University of British Columbia

IODINE

The occurrence of iodine deficiency in cardiovascular disease is frequent. The thyroid hormone deficiency on cardiovascular function can be characterized with decreased myocardial contractility and increased peripheral vascular resistance, as well as with the changes in lipid metabolism. A study done with 42 patients with cardiovascular disease were divided into 5 subgroups on the ground of the presence of hypertension, congestive heart failure, cardiomyopathy, coronary dysfunction, and arrhythmia. When urine concentrations were tested the most decreased urine iodine concentration was detected in the subgroups with arrhythmia and congestive heart failure. An elevated TSH level was found by 3 patients and elevation in lipid metabolism (cholesterol, triglyceride) associated with all subgroups without arrhythmia. The researchers concluded that iodine supplementation might prevent the worsening effect of iodine deficiency on cardiovascular disease.

Dr. Michael Donaldson, Research Director of the Hallelujah Diet, says, "Iodine stabilizes the heart rhythm, lowers serum cholesterol, lowers blood pressure, and is known to make the blood thinner as well, judging by longer clotting times seen by clinicians. Iodine is not only good for the cardiovascular system, it is vital. Sufficient iodine is needed for a stable rhythmic heartbeat. Iodine, directly or indirectly, can normalize serum cholesterol levels and normalize blood pressure. Iodine attaches to insulin receptors and improves glucose metabolism. Iodine and iodine-rich foods have long been used as a treatment for hypertension and cardiovascular disease; yet, modern randomized studies examining the effects of iodine on cardiovascular disease have not been carried out."

Clinical cardiovascular features of hypothyroidism include bradycardia, reduced cardiac output, increased pericardial and pleural effusions, increased diastolic blood pressure, and peripheral vasoconstriction. According to Dr. Stephen A. Hoption Cann, iodine deficiency can have deleterious effects on the cardiovascular system, and correspondingly, that a higher iodine intake may benefit cardiovascular function.

Adequate iodine is necessary for proper thyroid function. The heart is a target organ for thyroid hormones. Marked changes occur in cardiac function in patients with hypo- or hyperthyroidism.

In his newsletter *Health Alert* Dr. Bruce West says, "Iodine supplementation may be the missing link in a good percentage of heart arrhythmia cases, especially atrial fibrillation. The body needs adequate stores of iodine for the heart to beat smoothly. After close to a year now of using Iodine Fulfillment Therapy, I can attest to this fact. Most of the stubborn cases of cardiac arrhythmias and atrial fibrillation that we were unable to completely correct with our cardiac protocols have now been resolved with adequate supplies of iodine added to the protocol."

"Amazingly, while medicine shuns iodine therapy, their most popular anti-fibrillation drug, Amiodarone, actually is iodine in a more toxic, sustained-release form. This drug can produce a smooth heartbeat when the body has accumulated about 1,500 mgs of iodine—the exact amount of iodine retained by your body when iodine fulfillment is achieved by natural supplementation with Prolamine iodine. Unfortunately, Amiodarone is an extremely toxic form of iodine used by the medical profession. The side effects are often too great (and even life threatening) for most people to endure long enough to achieve a normal heartbeat. In addition, once you stop this drug, your original problem returns. Iodine therapy, on the other hand, fulfills the body's needs safely then maintains the smooth heartbeat with a low-maintenance dose," wrote Dr. West.

Dr. John Young in Tampa, Florida has been experimenting with a new process for reversing metabolic syndrome and Type 2 diabetes. Over the past 7 years he claims to have a success rate of 80 percent with over 100 diabetes patients. Dr. Young uses a combination of alkaline protein and minerals with a form of iodine that he says reverses the process in diabetes patients in eight to 12 weeks.

Dr. George Flechas has found that iodine can reduce the need for insulin in diabetic patients, using 50 to 100 mg of iodine per day. Of twelve patients, six were able to completely come off their medications with random glucose readings below 100 mg/dl and an HbA1cless than 5.8 (normal), and the other six were able to reduce the amount and/or number of medications needed to control their diabetes.

"Whole body sufficiency of iodine/iodide results in optimal cardiac functions," writes Dr. Guy Abraham. There is an epidemic of cardiac arrhythmias and atrial fibrillation in this country and Dr. Abraham is convinced that the medical iodine phobia has a great deal to do with this phenomenon. Adequate stores of iodine are necessary for a smooth heartbeat.

SELENIUM

Selenium (Se) is not only crucial when using iodine, but it addresses most directly the *Hun Hordes of Mercury* that are attacking heart tissues in massive amounts leading to cardiac arrest. What is not known by many is that mercury is a deadly cardiac poison whose best antidote is selenium—since they bind together making it easier for the body to remove the selenium-mercury compound. Magnesium of course is the *ultimate heart medicine*. Magnesium deficiency is directly correlated with most cardiovascular problems, including high blood pressure.

Selenium is absolutely essential in the age of mercury toxicity for it is the perfect antidote for mercury exposure. It is literally raining mercury all over the world but especially in the northern hemisphere. And of course with the dentists poisoning a world of patients with mercury dental amalgam and the doctors with their mercury laden vaccines, selenium is more important than most of us can imagine. One must remember that mercury strips the body of selenium, for the selenium stores get used up quickly because of its great affinity for mercury.

Selenium, an important antioxidant in the thyroid and involved in the metabolism of iodine-containing thyroid hormones, may play an interactive role in the development of these thyroid irregularities, and in turn, cardiovascular disease.

—Dr. Stephen Hoption Cann

Dr. Donaldson reminds us of the selenium iodine connection saying, "Another factor in how much iodine can be safely used depends on other possible mineral deficiencies. Selenium is very important for thyroid function. Selenium is part of the anti-oxidant enzyme glutathione peroxidase. Glutathione peroxidase in the thyroid helps quench free radicals produced by the enzyme thyroid peroxidase (which functions to organify iodide as it enters the thyroid). If high levels of iodide are present in the thyroid without sufficient amounts of glutathione peroxidase it causes free-radical damage to the thyroid, leading to autoimmune thyroid disease. Several of the enzymes that convert T4 into T3 also require selenium. Studies in Zaire have found that supplementing selenium and iodine deficient children with just selenium had adverse effects on thyroid function."

Selenium deficiency impairs thyroid hormone metabolism by inhibiting the synthesis and activity of the iodothyronine deiodinases, which convert thyroxine (T4) to the more metabolically active 3,3'-5 triiodothyronine (T3). In rats, concurrent selenium and iodine deficiency produces greater increases in thyroid weight and plasma thyrotrophin than iodine deficiency alone, indicating that a concurrent selenium deficiency could be a major determinant of the severity of iodine deficiency.

Later studies showed that serum T4 was maintained at control levels when both dietary iodine and selenium were low but not when iodine alone, or selenium alone, was low. Activity of thyroidal GSH-Px (erythrocyte glutathione peroxidase) was lowest in rats fed a diet containing high iodine and low selenium. The results suggested that high iodine intake, when selenium is deficient, may permit thyroid tissue damage as a result of low thyroidal GSH-Px activity during thyroid stimulation. A moderately low selenium intake normalized circulating T4 concentration in the presence of iodine deficiency.

Adequate selenium nutritional status may help protect against some of the neurological effects of iodine deficiency. Researchers involved in the Supplementation en Vitamines et Mineraux AntioXydants (SU.VI.MAX) study in France, which was designed to assess the effect of vitamin and mineral supplements on chronic disease risk, evaluated the relationship between goiter and selenium in a subset of this research population. Their findings suggest that selenium supplements may be protective against goiter. Selenium in the form of selenocysteine is an essential component of the family of the detoxifying enzymes glutathione peroxidase (Gpx) and of the iodothyronine selenodeiodinases that catalyze the extrathyroidal production of tri-iodothyronine (T(3)). Thus, Se deficiency may seriously influence the generation of free radicals, the conversion of thyroxine (T(4)) to T(3) and a thyroidal autoimmune process.

Recent studies concluded that a positive effect of Se on thyroidal autoimmune process was shown and indicated that high serum Se levels (>120 ug/l) may also influence the outcome of GD. (Graves disease). A recent study testing the various dosages of selenium confirmed that doses greater than 100 mcg of selenium (as L-selenomethionine) were required to maximize glutathione peroxidase activities in autoimmune thyroiditis.

Selenium is also essential for the production of estrogen sulfotranserfase which is the enzyme which breaks down estrogen. A deficiency of selenium can thus lead to excessive amounts of estrogen, which may depress thyroid function and also upset the progesterone-estrogen balance. Animal studies have shown that the addition of selenium supplementation will alleviate the effects of excess iodine intake. Iodine and selenium deficiencies must both be resolved for iodine treatment to be effective.

CONCLUSION

Iodine is critical in maintaining a healthy heart and selenium is involved in the metabolism of iodine containing hormones and therefore, is needed to combat cardiovascular disease. Iodine is also crucial in the prevention and treatment of cancer, which will be covered in the next chapter.

11. *Iodine Treats and Prevents Cancer*

In concert with its antioxidant and anti-inflammatory actions, iodine affects several molecular pathways that are part of differentiation and apoptosis in cells. Ongoing epidemiological evidence points to iodine's role in prevention and treatment of cancers through these effects.

High rates of goiter (iodine deficiency) correlates with higher rates of cancer mortality. This has been known for over 100 years especially for breast and stomach cancer. Other cancers associated with low iodine goiter conditions include prostate cancer, endometrial, ovarian, colorectal, and thyroid cancer.

Women with goiters (a visible, non-cancerous enlargement of the thyroid gland) owing to iodine deficiency have been found to have a three times greater incidence of breast cancer. A high intake of iodine is associated with a low incidence breast cancer, and a low intake with a high incidence of breast cancer.

—Dr. Donald Miller, Jr.

Cancer starts with iodine deficiencies just as it does with low oxygenation of tissues, with no one looking into the fact that low iodine and low oxygenation of tissues are directly related. Doctors are still scratching their heads wondering why cancer rates have been exploding, but do not pay attention to doctors like Brownstein who has seen over 90 percent deficiency rates among his patients and reports other doctors seeing the same.

Dr. Miller reports, "Health comparisons between the two countries are disturbing. The incidence of breast cancer in the U.S. is the highest in the world, and in Japan, until recently, the lowest. Japanese women who emi-grate from Japan or adopt a Western style diet have a higher rate of breast cancer compared with those that consume seaweed. Life expectancy in the U.S. is 77.85 years, 48th in 226 countries surveyed. It is 81.25 years in Japan, the highest of all industrialized countries and only slightly behind the five leaders—Andorra, Macau, San Marino, Singapore, and Hong Kong. The infant mortality rate in Japan is the lowest in the world, 3.5 deaths under age one per 1,000 live births, half the infant mortality rate in the United States."

Japanese women, who have one of the lowest breast cancer rates in the world, ingest more than 13 mg of iodine daily from seaweed without suffering any adverse consequences.

In addition to the thyroid and mammary glands, other tissues possess an iodine pump (the sodium/iodine symporter). Stomach mucosa, the sali-vary glands, and lactating mammary glands can concentrate iodine almost to the same degree as the thyroid gland (40-fold greater than its concentra-tion in blood). Other tissues that have this pump include the ovaries and the thymus gland, which is the seat of the adaptive immune system.

IODINE PREVENTS CANCERS

Dr. Brownstein clearly lays out what we would expect to find in iodine deficient individuals. When iodine is deficient nodules form in key organs leading to pre-cancerous conditions and then eventually to full-blown cancer. He says, "Iodine's main job is to maintain a normal architecture of those tissues. With iodine deficiency, the first thing that happens is you get cystic formation in the breasts, the ovaries, uterus, thyroid, prostate and, let's throw in the pancreas in here as well, which is also increasing at epi-demic rates—pancreatic cancer. Cysts start to form when iodine deficiency is there. If it goes on longer, they become nodular and hard. If it goes on longer, they become hyperplastic tissue, which is the precursor to cancer. I say that's the iodine deficiency continuum."

Brownstein continues, "The good thing about iodine is, iodine has apoptotic properties, meaning it can stop a cancer cell from just continually dividing, dividing, dividing until it kills somebody. Iodine can stop this continuum wherever it catches it and hopefully reverse it, but at least put the brakes on what is happening."

The earlier a cell is in its path toward an aggressive cancer the more likely it is to reverse course and go back to being healthy again. Therefore, for example, cells that are early precursors of cervical cancer are likely to revert. One study found that 60 percent of precancerous cervical cells, found with Pap tests, revert to normal within a year; 90 percent revert within three years.

IODINE TREATS CANCERS

Brownstein reports three cases of spontaneous regression of breast cancer after women take iodine supplementation in his iodine book. This should come as no surprise as a 2008 paper by Dr. Bernard A. Eskin showed that iodine actually altered gene expression in breast cancer cells, inducing programmed cell death.

Dr. Richard A. Kunin says, "Another organ that takes up iodine is the testicle. Proof of this fact is evident in the fact that treatment of thyroid cancer with RAI131 is sometimes followed by diminished or absent sperm counts and elevated pituitary gonadotropin hormone levels up to three and a half years later. Recovery also occurs but sterility is clearly a hazard of radioactive iodine treatment. Cancer is another hazard: One of my patients developed a testicular cancer fifteen years after radioactive iodine treatment for Grave's disease. His father had also had a testicular tumor (seminoma) so it would be prudent to avoid radioactive iodine therapy if one has such a history."

Dr. Brownstein has found in his research with high doses of iodine that cysts on the ovaries became smaller and began to disappear. He also found that libido in women and men increased and that is why painting the testicles with iodine helps with low libido and erectile dysfunction.

A 2003 study by Ling Zhang showed that molecular iodine caused lung cancer cells to undergo programmed cell death (apoptosis). Interestingly, a 1993 case report describes spontaneous remission of lung cancer in a patient incidentally treated with Amiodorone, which contains iodine (about 9 mg per day).

Iodine may also be affecting the binding of estrogen receptors to the steroid-binding element. Using breast cancer cells (MCF-7 cells), Stoddard and colleagues demonstrated that Lugol's solution (5 percent iodine/10 percent iodide) affected 43 genes involved cell cycle growth, proliferation, and differentiation. Many of the 43 genes are those upregulated by estrogens, implying that the Lugol's solution interfered with this action and had a net "antiestrogenic" effect on gene expression.

CANCER/FUNGUS THEORY

There are certain physical properties of cells that change, that make us call them cancerous. Tumor cells display a characteristic set of features that distinguish them from normal cells. All cancer cells acquire the ability to grow and divide in the absence of appropriate signals and/or in the presence of inhibitory signals. Acquired functional capabilities of cancer cells include:

- Evading apoptosis
- Insensitivity to antigrowth signals
- Limitless potential for replication
- Self-sufficiency in growth signals
- Sustained angiogenesis
- Tissue invasion and metastasis

Dr. Luke Curtis, MD, is reporting on research that deals with 27 lung "cancer" patients who were later diagnosed with lung "fungus" instead of lung cancer. "Fungal infection can present with clinical and radiological features that are indistinguishable from thoracic malignancy, such as lung nodules or masses." Doctors who diagnose lung cancer are unaware of the fact that cancer mimics fungal infections.

A medical textbook used to educate Johns Hopkins medical students in 1957, Clinical and Immunologic Aspects of Fungous Diseases, declared that many fungal conditions look exactly like cancer!

—Doug A. Kaufmann, The Germ That Causes Cancer

Fungus, which is the most powerful and the most organized micro-organism known, seems to be an extremely logical candidate as a cause of neoplastic proliferation, Dr. Tullio Simoncini says, "*Candida albicans* clearly emerges as the sole candidate for tumoral proliferation."

Cancer is a biologically-induced spore (fungus) transformation disease.

—Dr. Milton W. White

An entirely new way of looking at the relationship between cancer and fungus is seeing that cancer begins when the DNA from fungus and the DNA from our white blood cells merge to form a new hybrid "tumor, or sac." This hybrid attains a life of its own now, bypassing our immune defenses because it is 50 percent human, and therefore just enough to be recognized as "self."

Fungi are parasites whose mission is to invade a larger host.
Given a chance they will alter our body chemistries to suit their needs.

The white cells can end up protecting the fungus and its DNA as "friend" because it has been incorporated inside the macrophages effectively hiding the invader from our other immune defenses. Unfortunately, for us *fungal cells always become the dominant cells*. (See Chapter 4 for more on the Fungus/Cancer Theory.)

In their refutation of the theory of autoimmunity, Kaufman and Holland explain that in Type 1 diabetes it is entirely plausible that invading fungi have altered beta cells, remained undetected, yet set off the body's immune defense system, which is unable to destroy the offending fungi allowing them to continue to invade other beta cells and progressively lead to total destruction and a complete lack of insulin. The extremely manipulative ways that fungi work to ensure their own food supply is highly characteristic of their nature.

A recent Japanese study suggests that fungal mold toxins have the ability
to signal the beta cells in the pancreas to shut them off by killing them.

A.V. Constantini, MD, former head of the WHO Collaborating Center for Mycotoxins in Food has spent 20 years studying and collecting data on the role fungi and mycotoxins play in devastating diseases. In his research, he found a number of fungi that demonstrate specific toxicity to the pancreas.

When fungal colonization and mycotoxin contamination is maximal
one finds cancer growing and mestastizing at a maximal rate.

TREATING VIRUSES

There is not only one way to skin the cat (virus). Directly supporting the immune system through a number of natural means and replenishing Vitamin C faster than Ebola strips it from the body creating lightening Scurvy and massive hemorrhage is another. Hitting the body hard with glutathione and selenium is yet another potent and intelligent avenue of treatment that is not being pursued by the western medical establishment.

As mentioned in Chapter 4, when a cell becomes full of virus, it bursts, releasing the virus to infect other host cells. Certain viruses infect host cells by fusion with cellular membranes at low pH. These viruses are classified as "pH-dependent viruses." Fusion of viral and cellular membranes is pH dependent. "The plasma membrane of eukaryotic cells serves as a barrier against invading parasites and viruses. To infect a cell, viruses must be capable of transporting their genome and accessory proteins into the host cell, bypassing or modifying the barrier properties imposed by the plasma membrane. Entry into the host cells always involves a step of membrane fusion for enveloped animal viruses. Other enveloped viruses, such as orthomyxoviruses, alphaviruses or rhabdoviruses enter the cells by the endocytic pathway, and fusion depends on the acidification of the endosomal compartment. Fusion at the endosome level is triggered by conformational changes in viral glycoproteins induced by the low pH of this cellular compartment."

It has been suggested that the hepatitis C virus (HCV) infects host cells through a pH-dependent internalization mechanism. This HCVpp-mediated fusion was dependent on low pH, with a threshold of 6.3 and an optimum at about 5.5 (*See* Chapter 4). When pH drops to 6 or below, rapid fusion between the membranes of viruses and the liposomes occurs.

Induction of Poliovirus Entry by Exposure of the Cells to Low pH

In the case of a number of enveloped viruses and diphtheria toxin, the acidic vesicles can be bypassed if cells with surface-bound virus or toxin are exposed to low pH. Under these conditions, entry apparently occurs directly from the cell surface. Scientific investigation indicates that low pH is indeed required for the entry of poliovirus. The ability of cells to alter poliovirus in the presence of monensin was strongly increased at low pH. The main finding of one study is that a strain of poliovirus type 1 requires low pH for injection of its genome into the cytosol.

As it is with viral infections it is with cancer. The external pH of solid tumors is acidic as a consequence of increased metabolism of glucose and poor perfusion. Acid pH has been shown to stimulate tumor cell invasion and metastasis in vitro and in cells before tail vein injection in vivo.

Drugs that increase intracellular pH (alkalinity within the cell) have been shown to decrease infectivity of pH-dependent viruses. However pharmaceutical drugs that do this can provoke negative side effects. Sodium bicarbonate is the best way to increase pH in clinical emergency conditions and has been known as far back as the Spanish Flu pandemic of 1918 to save lives.

Increases of Carbon Dioxide and Bicarbonates Lead to Increased Oxygen

The most important factor in creating proper pH is increasing oxygen because no wastes or toxins can leave the body without first combining. with oxygen. The more alkaline you are, the more oxygen your fluids can hold and keep. Oxygen also buffers/oxidizes metabolic waste acids helping to keep you more alkaline. "The Secret of Life is both to feed and nourish the cells and let them flush their waste and toxins", according to Dr. Alexis Carrell, Nobel Prize recipient in 1912. Dr. Otto Warburg, also a Nobel Prize recipient, in 1931 and 1944, said, "If our internal environment was changed from an acidic oxygen deprived environment to an alkaline environment full of oxygen, viruses, bacteria, and fungus cannot live."

The position of the oxygen disassociation curve (ODC) is influenced directly by pH, core body temperature, and carbon dioxide pressure. According to Warburg, it is the increased amounts of carcinogens, toxicity, and pollution that cause cells to be unable to uptake oxygen efficiently. This is connected with over-acidity, which itself is created principally under low oxygen conditions.

According to Annelie Pompe, a prominent mountaineer and world-champion free diver, alkaline tissues can hold up to 20 times more oxygen than acidic ones. When our body cells and tissues are acidic (below pH of 6.5 to 7.0) they lose their ability to exchange oxygen and cancer cells love that.

CONCLUSION

As you learned in this chapter, iodine is a vital component in human bio-chemistry. It has antioxidant, antiseptic, antibacterial, and anti-inflammatory characteristics, which may singularly aid in the treatment of cancer. It is more and more being recognized to be anti-carcinogenic and have cell differentiation properties as well as being effective in triggering apoptosis (cancer cell death). The use of iodine for breast cancer treatment follows in Chapter 12.

12. *Iodine for Breast Cancer and Skin Cancer*

Breast cancer is the most common type of cancer in women and is the second leading cause of cancer death in women (after lung cancer). The American Cancer Society estimates that in 2017, about 252,710 new cases of invasive breast cancer and 63,410 new cases of breast carcinoma in situ (confined to the breast milk duct) in women were diagnosed—and 40,610 died from the disease.

Skin cancer rates have been on the rise for 30 years, despite decades of lectures about sunscreen. Skin cancer is the most common cancer in this country, with more young people having skin cancer than ever before. Nearly 5 million Americans are treated for the disease each year, and the incidence rate is up 300 percent from 1994. Indoor tanning alone is linked to 419,000 cases of skin cancer a year in the U.S. Though melanoma represents only a small percentage of diagnoses, it can spread fast and be lethal, and it's the most common form of cancer among young adults aged 25 to 29.

It is important to realize that many scientists believe viruses, fungi, and bacteria are all different stages of the microbe life cycle and are directly involved in all forms of cancer including skin and breast cancer. Therefore using iodine, an antifungal medicine, makes sense. As cited in Chapter 4, Dr. Simoncini theorizes that skin cancers are caused by the *Candida* fungus (see page 38). A significant number of cancer researchers have found evidence supporting the cancer fungus link (see Chapter 4) so using bicarbonate and iodine, both antifungal medicines, is beneficial.

BREAST CANCER

Dr. Sherrill Sellman's book, *What Women Must Know to Protect Their Daughters From Breast Cancer*, says, "Breast cancer will always be a tragedy that befalls a woman. It tears at the very fabric of a woman's life, rippling out to touch all those in her world. The fears, uncertainties, and pain are deeply and profoundly shared by family, friends, and co-workers. It is even a greater tragedy when young women are faced with this crisis because the tumors tend to be more aggressive. Young women also have to face the grim reality of a more advanced cancer at the time of diagnosis and higher mortality rates. Not one of them ever suspected, at their age, they would be become a breast cancer statistic. A breast cancer diagnosis always comes as a shock; no one ever expects it, especially young, vibrant, and seemingly healthy women."

Dr. Donald Miller, Jr., Professor Emeritus of Surgery at the University of Washington, writes, "The ductal cells in the breast, the ones most likely to become cancerous, are equipped with an iodine pump (the sodium iodine symporter, the same one that the thyroid gland has) to soak up this element." Miller points out, "Today 1 in 7 American women (almost 15 percent) will develop breast cancer during their lifetime. Thirty years ago, when iodine consumption was twice as high as it is now (480 µg a day) 1 in 20 women developed breast cancer. Iodine was used as a dough conditioner in making bread, and each slice of bread contained 0.14 mg of iodine. In 1980, bread makers started using bromide as a conditioner instead, which competes with iodine for absorption into the thyroid gland and other tissues in the body. Iodine was also more widely used in the dairy industry 30 years ago than it is now."

Breast cancer confronts women with the deepest issues of vulnerability and womanhood. The most common sexual side effects of breast removal stem from damage to a woman's feelings of attractiveness. In our culture, we are taught to view breasts as a basic part of beauty and femininity. If her breast has been removed, a woman may be insecure about whether her partner will accept her and find her sexually pleasing. Whatever does damage to a woman's vulnerabilities does damage to her sexuality.

Multiple Causes Of Breast Cancer

Doctors seldom know why one woman develops breast cancer and another does not, and most women who have breast cancer will never be able to pinpoint an exact cause. Breast cancer is the most common invasive cancer in females worldwide. It accounts for 16 percent of all female cancers and 22.9 percent of invasive cancers in women; 18.2 percent of all cancer deaths worldwide, including both males and females, are from breast cancer. Breast cancer is the most common major cancer in American women.

About 1 in 8 U.S. women (about 12.4 percent) will develop invasive breast cancer over the course of her lifetime. In 2018, an estimated 266,120 new cases of invasive breast cancer are expected to be diagnosed in women in the U.S., along with 63,960 new cases of non-invasive (in situ) breast cancer.

Dr. Brownstein says, "The chance of a woman having invasive breast cancer sometime during her life is now one in seven. The single most important nutrient to halt this progression is iodine. Inadequate breast iodine levels have been associated with the development of breast cancer in both animals and humans, while iodine supplementation has been shown to cause cancer cells to shift into apoptosis or programmed cell death. I have no doubt one of the reasons we are seeing such an epidemic of breast cancer is due to iodine deficiency."

Dr. Robert Thompson said, "I'm going to make a bold statement here: Iodine shortfalls coupled with bromine and other toxic halogens cause fibrocystic breast disease and breast cancer. Breast tissue contains the body's third highest concentrations of this essential mineral, so shortfalls in iodine needs have a highly negative impact on breast tissue. When you don't have enough iodine in your diet, or when you are iodine compromised because of exposure to the toxic halogens chlorine, fluorine, and bromine, the breast and thyroid compete for the little iodine that is available. The result is that the iodine supply in the thyroid and breasts is depleted, opening the door to thyroid related disorders, fibrocystic breast disease, and breast cancer."

Dr. Tina Kaczor reported that, "The first report of geographical regions with high rates of goiter having higher rates of cancer mortality was published in 1924. Ongoing epidemiological data has corroborated the association between goitrogenous regions and cancer incidence/mortality, particularly that of stomach cancer. Epidemiological evidence also suggests that thyroid disorders, particularly goiter, may be associated with breast cancer incidence and/or mortality. Other cancers associated with goitrogenic state include prostate cancer, endometrial, ovarian, colorectal, and thyroid cancer. It is not clear whether these associations are due to an underlying hypothyroid state, the presence of occult autoimmune processes, or iodine deficiency itself."

We can see that the medical establishment just does not want to look at radiation as the cause of breast cancer, nor do they want to tell women that by wearing their bras 24 hours per day they will have a 3 out of 4 chance of developing breast cancer. Women who wore bras more than 12 hour per day but not to bed, lower their risk to 1 out of 7. They also do not want to tell women what sexual and emotional stress can do their breasts. In *The Breast Journal*, we read an *Essay on Sexual Frustration as the Cause of Breast Cancer in Women: How Correlations and Cultural Blind Spots Conceal Causal Effects.*

We already know that depressed people suffer higher rates of cancer. They die more frequently from it than their happier peers. Individuals who are more depressed are 2.3 times more likely to die of cancer than their non-depressed counterparts are. Medicine recognizes that breast cancer patients with a history of traumatic or stressful life events have a two-fold increased risk of recurrence.

Perceptive doctors, who know how to listen to their patients, should be able to create a map of causes, a picture of inner disharmonies that lead to each woman's cancer. When it comes to breast cancer Dr. Nalini Chilkov says, "Cancer risk increases when the immune system is compromised by stress, loss of sleep, depression, inability to eat, poor nutrition. When a woman is traumatized by sexual violence and sexual assault, particularly if it was perpetrated by someone she trusted, such as her partner or a family member, her immune system will be compromised and her risk of many diseases, including cancer, will increase."

Risks

A woman's breasts are one of her most sensitive areas when it comes to cancers caused by radiation exposure. Dr. David Brownstein says, "Unfortunately, screening mammograms, used for nearly 30 years, have never been shown to alter breast cancer mortality. Moreover, to make matters worse, mammography exposes sensitive tissue to ionizing radiation, which actually causes cancer. A Norwegian study found that mammogram screening may reduce the risk of death from breast cancer by only 10 percent. Mette Kalager, M.D. and colleagues followed 40,075 women, screened and unscreened from 1996 through 2005."

Dr. Russell Blaylock says studies show mammograms actually increase a woman's risk of developing breast cancer from 1 to 3 percent per year, depending on the technique used. If women religiously undergo a mammogram every year for 10 years, they increase their risk from 10 to 30 percent. "By the age of 50, a full 45 percent of women will have cancer cells in their breasts. This does not mean that all these women will develop breast cancer, because in most women these cancer cells remain dormant. What it does mean is that, if you are one of these 45 percent of women, you are at high risk of spurring these cancer cells to full activity (when exposing their breasts to radiation)."

Breast cancer survivors of chemotherapy are facing increased risk of heart disease; so much so that at least some doctors are debating if it's time to abandon a chemotherapy mainstay. Drugs called anthracyclines are a breast chemo staple despite the well-known risk: They weaken women's hearts. "In the process of curing their breast cancer, we've exposed them to some pretty nasty things. And it's not just one nasty thing, it's a sequence of nasty things," explains Dr. Pamela Douglas, a Duke University cardiologist. Iodine on the other hand strengthens women's hearts.

Dr. Michael Friedman says, "Women are particularly at risk due to environmental agents depleting iodine reserves and other agents exposing them to radioactive I-131. After the thyroid gland, the distal portions of the human mammary glands are the heaviest users/concentrators of iodine in tissue. Iodine is readily incorporated into the tissues surrounding the mammary nipples and is essential for the maintenance of healthy functioning breast tissue. The radioactive decay of I-131 in breast tissue may be a significant factor in the initiation and progression of both breast cancer and some types of breast nodules."

Treatments

A breast-cancer diagnosis is a stressful and emotional experience. Many women feel as if they have to act quickly, having been trained to think that treating cancer as soon and as aggressively as possible is ideal. It is not. Doctors know that even with invasive cancers women do not need to be treated within days or even weeks of a diagnosis. There is enough time to try out much safer treatments like iodine and other natural agents like hemp oil, sodium bicarbonate, slow breathing, selenium, and other medicinals that belong in a complete cancer protocol.

Breast-cancer treatments may be effective at treating many tumors, but they come with a price. In the latest study on the side effects of these treatments, published in the journal *Cancer,* researchers led by Christopher Friese at the University of Michigan say that 42 percent of women who were treated for breast cancer reported severe side effects. These included nausea or vomiting, diarrhea, constipation, pain, swelling in the arms, shortness of breath, and skin irritation around the breasts during the seven months after diagnosis and following treatment with surgery, chemotherapy, or radiation.

Dr. David Derry said, "Lugol's solution is an iodine-in-water solution used by the medical profession for 200 years. One drop (6.5 mg per drop) of Lugol's daily in water, orange juice, or milk will gradually eliminate the first phase of the cancer development namely fibrocystic disease of the breast so no new cancers can start. It also will kill abnormal cells floating around in the body at remote sites from the original cancer. This approach appears to work for prostate cancer as prostate cancer is similar to breast cancer in many respects. Indeed, it likely will help with most cancers. Also higher doses of iodine are required for inflammatory breast cancer. As well we know that large doses of intravenous iodine are harmless which makes one wonder what effect this would have on cancer growth."

Iodine to the Rescue

High intake of iodine is associated with a lower risk of breast cancer. Women with a history of low iodine levels (hypothyroidism) face a significantly higher risk of developing liver cancer. Researchers led by Manal Hassan of Anderson Cancer Center at the University of Texas concluded that this finding suggested a clinical association between hypothyroidism and hepatitis C, which is contributing to the country's rising rate of liver cancer.

The first thing that happens to a woman when she develops an iodine deficiency is a problem with her reproductive organs; breast deformation, and general calcification. Dr. David Miller says that, "Iodine is needed in microgram amounts for the thyroid; milligram amounts for breast and other tissues, and can be used therapeutically in gram amounts."

In addition to fixing almost all cases of breast cysts, iodine also has a remarkable healing effect on ovarian cysts," says Dr. Robert Rowen. Though few know it, swollen ovaries is a condition analogous to goiter, when the thyroid swells in response to iodine deficiency. In the case of Polycystic Ovary Syndrome (PCOS), the starvation of the ovaries causes them to become cystic, swollen, and eventually unable to regulate the synthesis of their hormones leading to imbalances and infertility.

Iodine is an answer to breast cancer and cancer in general, and when used with other agents in the context of a full protocol can replace toxic chemotherapy. Today there is a growing awareness that many breast cancer patients each year could be spared chemotherapy without hurting their chances for survival. "We are backing off on chemotherapy and using chemotherapy more selectively" in certain women, said Dr. Eric Winer of the Dana-Farber Cancer Institute in Boston.

Fibrocystic Breast Disease

Women with fibrocystic breasts have bumpy, lumpy breasts that may have hardened areas. Ropy scar-like tissue or cysts and lumps characterize fibrocystic breast disease. Many women have both symptoms and some have nipple discharge as well. They are sometimes painful. Pain has been linked to hormone fluctuations during the menstrual cycle (lumps and bumps generally change throughout a woman's menstrual cycle), caffeine intake, and the use of oral contraceptives, but rarely is magnesium or iodine mentioned.

This condition has become so common that some doctors argue it is not a disease at all. More than half of all women experience fibrocystic breasts and cyclic breast tenderness at some point in their lives, and there is no surprise when you consider that over 90 percent of women are both iodine and magnesium deficient.

Russian studies investigating fibrocystic breast disease (FBD) discovered that the greater the iodine deficiency the greater the number of cysts in the ovaries. Since 1928, the iodine concentration in the ovary has been known to be higher than in every other organ except the thyroid.

Iodine's role in maintaining the health of breast tissue is suggested by its therapeutic effects on benign breast conditions. In a publication reviewing three clinical trials of varied designs, molecular iodine reduced fibrocystic signs/symptoms while iodide (I-) was less effective and affected thyroidal function more readily.

Dr. Jeffrey Dach writes about *The Iodine Crisis*, "If you are a woman diagnosed with fibrocystic breast disease or breast cancer, you need to read this book [*The Iodine Crisis* by Lynne Farrow]. If you are a woman who undergoes repeated breast biopsies or breast cyst aspirations, then you need to read this book. If you are a breast cancer survivor, then you need to read this book." Iodine is essential for healthy breasts and healthy children that feed off mother's milk. The role of concentrating iodine in lactating mammary tissue is clearly to provide necessary iodine to the developing child. With all the suffering women are facing with breast disease, you would think doctors would pay attention to iodine and bring it back into focus.

A review of three clinical studies using sodium iodide, protein-bound iodide, and molecular iodine showed clinical improvements in FBD of 70 percent, 40 percent, and 72 percent, respectively (Ghent et al. 1993).

Paget Disease

Paget disease of the breast (also known as Paget disease of the nipple and mammary Paget disease) is a rare type of cancer involving the skin of the nipple and, usually, the darker circle of skin around it, which is called the areola. Most people with Paget disease of the breast also have one or more tumors inside the same breast. These breast tumors are either ductal carcinoma in situ or invasive breast cancer.

What are the symptoms?

Paget Disease:
A Case Study

In November, a rare kind of breast cancer was found. A lady developed a rash on her breast, similar to that of young mothers who are nursing. Because her mammogram had been clear, the doctor treated her with antibiotics for infections. After 2 rounds, it continued to get worse, so her doctor sent her for another mammogram. This time it showed a mass. A biopsy found a fast growing malignancy. Chemo was started in order to shrink the growth; then a mastectomy was performed; then a full round of chemo; then radiation. After about 9 months of intense treatment, she was given a clean bill of health. She had one year of living each day to its fullest. Then the cancer returned to the liver area. She took 4 treatments and decided that she wanted quality of life, not the after-effects of chemo. She had 5 great months and she planned each detail of the final days. After a few days of needing morphine, she died.

This woman left this message to be delivered to women everywhere:

- A persistent redness, oozing, and crusting of your nipple causing it to itch and burn (in the case study below, it did not itch or burn much, and had no oozing, but it did have a crust along the outer edge on one side).

- A sore on your nipple that will not heal. (Mine was on the aureole area with a whitish thick looking area in center of nipple).

- Usually only one nipple is affected.

Breast Cancer Treatments Iodine with Sodium Bicarbonate

In the case of breast cancer Dr. Simoncini says, "In the presence of a tumor of large dimensions, before performing the treatment with iodine solution, it is necessary to perform a cycle of subcutaneous infiltrations with sodium bicarbonate at 5 percent under the lesion for the purpose of liberating the tissue from the possible invasion of the deep planes and of the basal lamina. If this is not done, we risk that the fungus, once destroyed at a superficial level, will defend itself by trespassing into those levels where a conclusive action of the iodine solution is impossible."

Women, *please* be alert to anything that is not normal, and be persistent in getting help as soon as possible. Paget disease of the nipple: This is a rare form of breast cancer, and is on the outside of the breast, on the nipple and aureole. It appeared as a rash, which later became a lesion with a crusty outer edge. I would not have ever suspected it to be breast cancer, but it was. My nipple never seemed any different to me, but the rash bothered me, so I went to the doctor for that. Sometimes, it itched and was sore, but other than that it didn't bother me. It was just ugly and a nuisance, and could not be cleared up with all the creams prescribed by my doctor and dermatologist for the dermatitis on my eyes just prior to this outbreak. They seemed a little concerned but did not warn me it could be cancerous.

Now, I suspect not many women out there know a lesion or rash on the nipple or aureole can be breast cancer. (Mine started out as a single red pimple on the aureole. One of the biggest problems with Paget disease of the nipple is that the symptoms appear to be harmless. It is frequently thought to be a skin inflammation or infection, leading to unfortunate delays in detection and care.)

"In cases where the tumor has invaded a coetaneous-mucous transitional zone like the anus, eyelids, vagina or mouth, it is necessary to perform a preliminary treatment of the mucous area with bicarbonate and then, after the elimination of the colonies existing there, proceed to treat the cutis with iodine solution. It is appropriate to highlight that the same type of therapy is to be applied also to psoriasis and to the known fungi afflictions. In fact, the difference between coetaneous mycosis, psoriases, and tumors consists only of a variation of aggressiveness and thus of depth of rooting, since the causal agent is always the same: a fungus. Sometimes for the therapy, other corrosive salts can be used in function of the location in the body." Meaning the deeper the cancer the more one needs to rely on injected and bicarbonate IVs and other systemic approaches to treatment like oral iodine.

Caution is always necessary when treating with iodine, because iodine can be very caustic on the skin sometimes, we can use transdermal iodine to saturate breast tissue to treat breast cancer. What Simoncini did not recognize is that we can also saturate the tissues from within with the oral intake of iodine thus combining oral with transdermal.

Other Recommendations

In my Natural Allopathic protocol, instead of IV infusions of bicarbonate, we treat intensively with oral and transdermal (baths) bicarbonate. Other topical treatments to the breasts can and should include magnesium oil massaged into the breasts, clay packs, slow breathing, and even infrared treatments. In the future, we will see sound waves used to heat the tissues to the point where cancer cells cannot survive but normal healthy cells do.

I recommend infrared sauna, specifically the Thermal Life and Transcend Far Infrared saunas from High Tech Health for detox of heavy metals because most cancer patients have heavy metals. Though I heavily recommend Biomats for all night infrared treatments to raise body temperature, comfort, and pain, here in Brazil I have built my own sauna because with saunas one sweats profusely and this carries out toxins.

SKIN CANCER

Skin cancer is the most commonly diagnosed cancer. Over one million cases are diagnosed each year, with more young people having skin cancer than ever before. Skin cancer can be categorized into two main types based on which kind of malignant skin cell it comes from (see Figure 13.1), non-melamoma skin cancer and malignant melanoma. Non-melanoma skin cancer is the most common type of cancer among men and women.

The most common types of skin cancer include:

- Basal cell

- Squamous cell

- Melanoma

Other rare types of skin cancer include keratoacanthomas, Merkel cell carcinoma, skin lymphoma, Kaposi sarcoma, skin adnexal tumors, and sarcomas. These are all non-melanoma types.

Basal Cell

More than 4 million cases of basal cell carcinoma are diagnosed in the U.S. every year, the most frequently occurring cancer. Basal cell carcinomas are lesions or growths that appear in the skin's basal cells. They arise in the outermost layer of the skin.

It often appears as a painless raised area of skin. They may appear as open sores, red patches, pink growths, shiny bumps, or scars and are usually caused by a combination of long-term and occasional sun exposure.

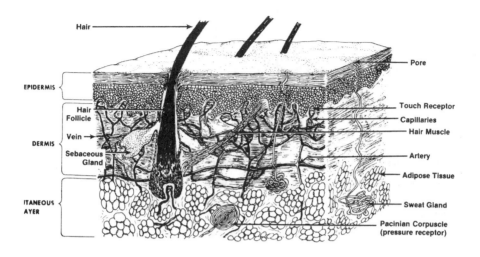

Figure 12.1. Types of Cancerous Skin Cells

Usually, the basal cell carcinoma will appear on parts of the body that are excessively exposed to the sun—especially the face, ears, neck, scalp, shoulders, and back. However, on rare occasions, lesions will develop on unexposed areas.

Squamous Cell

Squamous cell canrcinoma is the second most common skin cancer with more than one million cases occurring each year. It is a fast growth of abnormal cells found in the sequamous cells, the cells that make up the tissue that forms the surface of the skin's lining. They usually appear as rough, scaly patches of skin and may ooze blood if scratched or scraped and crusting may appear. They may materialize as open sores or warts.

Chronic infection and skin inflammation may also trigger this type of skin cancer. People who are fair skinned and have a history of substantial sun exposure are most at risk. They appear more frequently in men than in women.

Melanoma

Although melanoma is not the most common of the skin cancers, it is a dangerous type of skin cancer and has the most fatal results. If not diagnosed and treated at the early stages, it can advance and spread to other parts of the body where it is difficult to treat and can result in death.

Generally melanomas occur in the skin, however they may appear in the mouth, eyes, or intestines. In women they most commonly appear on the legs, while in men on the back. Melamoma appears more often in men than in women.

Once again, extended exposure to the sun may be the culprit in triggering this type of cancer, but genetics also plays an important role.

Treating with Iodine

Iodine is crucial in treating skin cancer, used orally and topically. It is also effective in treating potential cancer spots. Iodine applied to suspicious skin lesions can eliminate the risk of skin cancer. Apply to the affected area multiple times per day, alternating with sodium bicarbonate applications.

Most doctors are surprised when they hear oncologist Dr. Tullio Simoncini state, "Every tumour of the skin can be completely removed with Iodine Tincture 7 percent, brushed many times (10 to 20) once a day. When the crust is formed, don't take it away, but treat the area continuously and wait until it falls without any other intervention except the Iodine tincture. When the crust falls down the third time, the patient is healed."

Dr. Simoncini explains:

For epithileomas, basaliomas, and melanomas, the treatment to choose is iodine solution at seven percent as it is capable of precipitating the proteins of the body of the fungus and destroying them completely in a short time. If the lesions are fairly small, they must be painted with the solution 10–20–30 times twice a day for five days and then once for another ten days so that they become very dark. When the scar is formed and it is higher than the epidermic plane, it is necessary to continue to paint under and above it, even if at first a strong pain is sensed.

Keep in mind that any sore or lesion that refuses to heal over time should be regarded with suspicion and brought to the attention of your physician.

Tinctures of iodine are not suitable for oral ingestion and should be used transdermally only. Many iodine products are marked "not for oral ingestion" and one must heed this caution.

Dr. Simoncini has indicated that with iodine treatments for skin cancers that one should *never* disturb or pick or scrape off the scab that forms over the spot treated. Doing so will spread the fungus, the scab *must* be allowed to fall off all on its own, even if only hanging by a thread.

Iodine is available in every pharmacy in the world. However, the common inexpensive form found there cannot be taken orally, though it can be used for skin infections and skin cancer as well as systemic supplementation by getting in moderate dosages through the skin.

CONCLUSION

Women would have a lower incidence of cancer and fibrocystic disease of the breast if they consumed more iodine and other minerals like magnesium, selenium, and zinc. A decrease in iodine intake coupled with an increased consumption of competing halogens, fluoride, and bromide, has created an epidemic of iodine deficiency in America and this seems to be in part responsible for skyrocketing rates of breast cancer. It makes total sense that iodine, one of the nutrients that when deficient leads to breast cancer, would also help to cure it.

Most cases of skin cancer are easily treated with simple procedures. Using iodine as a precaution and treatment provides an uninviting environment for cancer cells to grow. It wipes out cancer cells, removes abnormal cells, kills viruses, and neutralizes toxins. Treating infectious diseases in children is covered in the chapter that follows.

13. Pediatric Iodine

Antibiotics have been overused and now they can be dangerous and ineffective against a generation of superbugs they helped create, see Chapter 4. Treatment with iodine when infections threaten may be a more effective field of medicine.

Infections cause child deaths. Iodine can save many of these children's lives. Iodine can save lives. More than two-thirds of the estimated 8.8 million deaths in children under the age of five worldwide in 2008 were caused by infectious diseases according to a study on behalf of the World Health Organization and the United Nations Children's Fund (UNICEF). The study, published in *The Lancet* found that infectious diseases caused 68 percent of deaths in under fives, led by pneumonia (18 percent, 1.58 million children), diarrhea (15 percent, 1.34 million) and malaria (8 percent, 0.73 million).

According to several studies, obstetricians and gynecologists write 2,645,000 antibiotic prescriptions every week. Internists prescribe 1,416,000 per week. This works out to 211,172,000 prescriptions annually in the United States, just for these two specialties. Pediatricians prescribe over $500 million worth of antibiotics annually just for one condition, ear infections. Yet topical povidone iodine (PVP-I) is as effective as topical ciprofloxacin, with a superior advantage of having no in vitro drug resistance and the added benefit of reduced cost of treatment.

EFFECTS OF PEDIATRIC ANTIOBIOTICS/VACCINES

Despite the growing evidence of a link between mercury and neurological disorders, such as autism, attention deficit disorder, language delay, and learning difficulties, which are being reported on a worldwide basis to be rising dramatically, the Institute of Medicine (IOM) and the CDC, and a long string of other medical organizations are certifying mercury, one of the most toxic chemicals known to man, as being absolutely safe for use in vaccines. And they continue to do that even as they alert the public to a pandemic that has one child in 166 being diagnosed with autism spectrum disorders and as many as one in six children diagnosed with a developmental disorder and/or with behavior problems.

By replacing vaccines and antibiotics with iodine, we only scratch the surface of the problems these medical practices create for children and their mothers. Medical scientists at Arizona State University tell us that antibiotic use is known to almost completely inhibit excretion of mercury in rats due to alteration of gut flora. The actual cost of not using iodine and instead using antibiotics goes beyond the creation of antibiotic resistant infections; it directly leads to increased rates of autism through mercury poisoning.

Mercury in Vaccines

Nowhere in the world of medicine do things get as ugly as in the vaccine loaded with mercury story and the same goes with dentistry, which packs mercury into peoples and children's mouths only inches from their brains. "Autism is upon us because it's the outcome of the 50-year experiment of dousing every living being with an overload of toxic substances, including vaccines," writes Dr. Gregory Ellis.

America's largest organization for pediatricians is strongly objecting to a proposal by the United Nations to ban a mercury-containing preservative from the world's vaccine supply. In a brief statement published online in *Pediatrics,* the academy supported the recommendations drafted by the WHO's Strategic Advisory Group of Experts (SAGE) on immunization at an April meeting that ignores all the science that suggests that the neurological poison thimerosal is dangerous, more dangerous than if they put lead in the vaccine instead.

---

*Thimerosal is one of the most toxic compounds I know of,
I can't think of anything that I know of that is more lethal.*
—Dr. Boyd Haley, University of Kentucky, Professor of Chemistry

---

Dr. Richard Halvorsen, author of the book, *The Truth About Vaccines,* said: "Thimerosal is an extremely toxic substance and a known poison to the brain. There is enough convincing evidence linking thimerosal with developmental disorders and learning problems in individual children to warrant its removal from any childhood vaccine."

Doctors, dentists, and nurses need to make their patients aware of the availability of mercury-free vaccines and the dangers of mercury-based products: Amalgam fillings, which are 50 percent mercury, and thimerosal used in the manufacture and preservation of vaccines, which is 50 percent mercury by weight. Mercury has been appropriately removed from most other medical products except these, for it is one of the most toxic and dangerous elements known to mankind.

Higher use of oral antibiotics, in children destined to contract autism, may have reduced their ability to excrete mercury. Higher usage of oral antibiotics in infancy may also partially explain the high incidence of chronic gastrointestinal problems in individuals with autism.

Hannah's Story

"My daughter, who had been completely normal until getting nine vaccinations in one day, was suddenly no longer there," said Terry P., mother of 9-year-old Hannah. Hannah P. appeared to be like many children. At 19 months, her pediatrician noted she was "alert and active" and "spoke well." At that same visit, she got five shots—nine doses of vaccines. She almost immediately developed fever, seizures, and severe health problems. Eight years later, the government has quietly conceded that vaccines aggravated a cell disorder nobody knew Hannah had, leaving her with permanent brain damage and autistic-like symptoms. Hannah was described as normal, happy, and precocious in her first 18 months.

In 2002, Hannah's parents filed an autism claim in federal vaccine court. Five years later, the government settled the case before trial and had it sealed. It's taken more than 2 years for both sides to agree on how much Hannah will be compensated for her injuries.

The first court award in a vaccine-autism claim was a big one. Hannah P. will receive more than $1.5 million for her life care, lost earnings, and pain and suffering for the first year alone. In addition to the first year, the family will receive more than $500,000 per year to pay for Hannah's care. Those familiar with the case believe the compensation could easily amount to $20 million over the child's lifetime

Yeast Overgrowth

Many pediatricians are unaware of lasting adverse effects caused by routinely prescribed antibiotics. Antibiotic therapy for minor colds and runny noses is a common practice. Antibiotics, such as tetracycline, can greatly increase yeast in the colon after only a few days.

The extensive use of antibiotics will make the condition of Candida much worse because it reduces heavy metal excretion.

Normally, *Candida albicans* lives peacefully in our intestines and elsewhere, in harmony with other flora that keep the yeast in check. Take an antibiotic and all this changes. By suppressing the normal flora, *Candida* takes over and problems begin. In its mild form the result is diarrhea or a yeast infection.

Dr. Elmer Cranton says that, "Yeast overgrowth is partly iatrogenic (caused by the medical profession) and can be caused by antibiotics and cortisone medications. A diet high in sugar also promotes overgrowth of yeast. A highly refined diet common in industrialized nations not only promotes growth of yeast, but is also deficient in many of the essential vitamins and minerals needed by the immune system. Chemical colorings, flavorings, preservatives, stabilizers, emulsifiers, etc., add more to stress on the immune system."

Children with autism had significantly (2.1-fold) higher levels of mercury in their baby teeth but similar levels of lead and similar levels of zinc. Children with autism also had significantly higher usage of oral antibiotics during their first 12 to 36 months of life.
—Journal of Toxicology and Environmental Health, 2007

Reporting in the July 11, 2007 issue of the *Journal of the American Medical Association*, researchers say the use of antibiotics boosts risks for drug resistance while doing nothing to shield kids from future urinary tract infections (UTIs). Prior use of antibiotics to prevent infection did boost the likelihood of developing a drug-resistant infection by nearly 7.5 times.

Many physicians seem to be unaware that birth control pills comprised of the hormones estrogen and progesterone can make the body more susceptible to fungal infections. If antibiotics are prescribed, it acts as a double whammy to ensuring a fungal infection will take hold by diminishing the protective bacteria in the intestines. Many pregnant women seek medical treatment for minor problems and are indiscriminately given antibiotics, which begins a long decline into problems. In many places in the world they still give mercury containing Hep B shots at birth even though Hepatitis B is not a childhood disease.

In 2005 a study the antibiotic Augmentin TM has been implicated in the formation of autism. The study strongly suggests the possibility of ammonia poisoning as a result of young children taking Augmentin. Augmentin has been given to children since the late 1980's for bacterial infections.

Autism

Antibiotics may be to blame for hundreds of children developing autism after having the controversial MMR (Measles-Mumps-Rubella) jab, which is not even controversial any more. It is just a bad vaccine based on wrong assumptions. Just recently the measles virus was declared by a German high court not even to exist, so what is in this dangerous vaccine is anyone's guess.

More than two-thirds of youngsters with the condition received four or more antibiotics in their first year, a British survey has revealed. It is thought the drugs weakened their immune systems, leaving them unable to withstand the impact of the triple jab.

Antibiotics are mostly derived from fungi and are therefore classified as mycotoxins. Mycotoxins are poisons.

New research shows a troubling correlation between a woman's thyroid function and her child's risk for autism. When "mothers had very low levels of thyroid hormone early in pregnancy the chance of having a kid with autism was multiplied by 4; very seldom we see these strength of association." A study published in the August issue of the *Annals of Neurology* brings crucial attention to iodine supplementation for pregnant women.

IODINE DEFICIENCY AFFECTS BRAIN DEVELOPMENT

Dr. Gustavo Roman, with the Houston Methodist Neurological Institute and researchers in the Netherlands, studied thousands of pregnant Dutch women and found a lack of iodine in their diets affected fetal brain development. "I think for the first time we have the possibility of finding an explanation of the problem, but most importantly we have a way of preventing this from happening," says Dr. Roman.

"I think it's very important that women of reproductive age measure the amount of iodine in the urine it's a very simple test and if the levels are low they need to go back to using iodized salt to prevent this from happening," concludes Roman. The problem with his suggestion is that there is little iodine in iodized salt and what is there evaporates rapidly when sitting on the table leaving nothing to absorb.

Insufficient maternal iodine during pregnancy can result
in a permanently lowered IQ as well as thyroid problems.
—Dr. David Brownstein

Doctors have consistently found in autism a combination of conditions, including severe intestinal dysbiosis, systemic fungal and viral infections, mineral deficiencies, abnormal serotonin levels, and an abundance of toxic materials, including pesticides, mercury, and other heavy metals. Autistic children are suffering from a heavy metal instigated gut and brain infections that create neurological dysfunctions. A fungal infection in the body of an expecting mother can become more acute as blood sugar levels naturally go up. All infections in the mother's blood are passed to her baby.

The *New York Times* reported that a new study of twins suggests that environmental factors, including conditions in the womb, may be at least as important as genes in causing autism. Mathematical modeling suggested that only 38 percent of the cases in the study could be attributed to genetic factors, whereas environmental factors appeared to be at work in 58 percent of the cases.

TREATING WITH IODINE

The minimum number of iodine molecules required to destroy one bacterium varies with the species. For H. influenzae it was calculated to be 15,000 molecules of iodine per cell. When bacteria are treated with iodine, the inorganic phosphate uptake and oxygen consumption by the cells immediately ceases.

Iodine is an excellent microbicide with a broad range of action that includes almost all of the important health-related microorganisms, such as enteric bacteria, enteric viruses, bacterial viruses, fungi and protozoan cysts.

Iodine is by far the best antibiotic, antiviral, and antiseptic of all time.

—Dr. David Derry

The thyroid gland is unable to differentiate between regular iodine and radioactive iodine and will uptake whatever chemical form it is presented with especially when one is already iodine deficient. The negative health consequences of radioactive iodine target the sensitive populations of the pregnant, unborn babies, and children up to 10 years of age most aggressively. If radioactive iodine is inhaled or ingested, it lingers in the body wherein it emits radioactive energy that results in internal damage mainly to the thyroid and parathyroid glands.

Newborn babies will uptake iodine at rates 16 times higher than adults do. Infants under the age of one have an 8 times higher uptake than adults. Five-year-old children have 4 times the adult uptake rate. Pregnant mothers have increased thyroid uptake, most noted in the first trimester. The unborn have an increased thyroid uptake in the second and third trimester of pregnancy. Nursing mothers can secrete 25 percent of iodine reserves to their babies.

CONCLUSION

Sufficient amounts of iodine are critical for thyroid hormone production, which is necessary for normal neurodevelopment during pregnancy and early childhood. The medical community needs to focus on the importance of iodine sufficiency, an issue that directly affects the well-being and neurodevelopment of children. In reading this chapter we can conclude that iodine should never have been replaced with antibiotics, which in the long run have hurt our children.

Conclusion

Our bodies are truly amazing works of nature. The systems that carry on our life processes within us were designed to be in balance with our environment. The problem, however, is that our environment has changed greatly. And beyond just the weather and the air, is the food we consume. We are no longer hunters and gathers living on instinct for our food and survival. For the most part, we are a "civilized" people no longer worried about where our next meal will come from. And that may be the very root of so many of our health problems.

We take for granted that we are getting all the nutrients—vitamins and mineral—from our daily diets, however that is far from the truth. In many cases, the foods we eat may in fact lack the very nutrients that they are known for. Our agricultural revolution has allowed farmers to grow their crops on played out soil through the "magic of chemistry." So while our food products look great, they may no longer contain the very elements meant to sustain us. This book is, in fact, a reflection of this growing problem. For the vast majority of our population, iodine appears to be a missing element in our food chain. Ninety percent of us are iodine deficient, and because of this we are subject to a number of terrible illnesses—as we have pointed out throughout this book.

The bigger problem for us is that many of these health issues can go undetected for years, and when their symptoms finally appear, they go untreated—because too few health practiners bother to test for iodine-based causes. In this book I have tried to focus on some of the major issues related to this problem, however there are a number of other problems I have not covered. My hope is by now you have come to understand just how important iodine is in relationship to maintaining good health. If you have not checked to see whether you are one of the millions of people who lack iodine in your body, now is the time to get tested. If you are suffering from one of the problems you have read about in this book, make sure you ask your healthcare provider about looking into it. And if he or she doesn't know anything about it, show them the book.

The bottom line is that you need to share responsibility for your state of health. The more information you have, the better informed decisions you will be able to make. And don't be afraid to double check the facts. Conflicting information abounds everywhere. However, if you take the right path and you see your health problem improve or completely clear up, you'll know if you've made the right choice.

Wishing you the best of health.

References

Abraham, G. "The Bioavailability of Iodine Applied to the Skin." http://www.optimox.com/iodine-study-20#1.

Abraham, GE. "The historical background of the iodine project." *The Original Internist* 2005;12(2):57–66.

Aceves, C, et al. "The extrathyronine actions of iodine as antioxidant, apoptotic, and differentiation factor in various tissues." *Thyroid* 2013:23:938–946.

Adams, JB, et al. "Mercury, lead, and zinc in baby teeth of children with autism versus controls." *J Toxicol Environ Health* 2007;70(12):1046–1051.

Arthur, JR, Nicol, F, Beckett, GJ. "The role of selenium in thyroid hormone metabolism and effects of selenium deficiency on thyroid hormone and iodine metabolism." *Biol Trace Elem Res* 1992;33:37–42.

Asayama, K, Kato, K. "Oxidative Muscular Injury and Its Relevance to Hyperthyroidism." *Free Radic Biol Med* 1999;8(3):293–303.

Bavari, S, et al. "Lipid Raft Microdomains: A Gateway for Compartmentalized Trafficking of Ebola and Marburg Viruses." *The Journal of Experimental Medicine* 2005;195(5):593–602.

Berking, S, et al. "A newly discovered oxidant defence system and its involvement in the development of Aurelia aurita (Scyphozoa, Cnidaria): reactive oxygen species and elemental iodine control medusa formation." *Int J Dev Biol* 2005;49:969–976.

Cann, S. "Hypothesis: Dietary Iodine Intake in the Etiology of Cardiovascular Disease." *J Am Coll Nutr* 2006;25(1):1–11.

Center for Veterinary Medicine. "The Human Health Impact of Fluoroquinolone-Resistant Campylobacter Attributed to the Consumption of Chicken." Washington, DC: Food and Drug Administration, 2000.

Chakrabarti, S, Fombonne, E. "Pervasive developmental disorders in preschool children." *JAMA* 2001;285:3093–3099.

Cheeke, PR. *Natural Toxicants in Feeds, Forages and Poisonous Plants.* Danville, IL: Interstate Publishers Inc., 1998.

Cobra, et al. "Infant Survival Is Improved by Oral Iodine Supplementation." *The Journal of Nutrition* 1997;127(4):574–578.

Colin, C, et al. "The brown algal kelp Laminaria digitata features distinct bromoperoxidase and iodoperoxidase activities." *J Biol Chem* 2003;278:23545–52.

Connolly, CP, et al. "Different Tissue Responses for Iodine and Iodide in Rat Thyroid and Mammary Glands." *Bio Trace Elem Res* 1995;49(1):9–19.

Cunnane, SC. *Survival of the Fattest: The Key to Human Brain Evolution.* Singapore: World Scientific Publishing Company, 2005.

Danzi, S, Klein, I. "Thyroid hormone and the cardiovascular system." *Minerva Endocrinol* 2004;29(3):139–150.

Da Poian, AT, et al. "Viral membrane fusion: is glycoprotein G of rhabdoviruses a representative of a new class of viral fusion proteins?" *Braz J Med Biol Res* 2005;38(6).

Derry, DM. *Breast Cancer and Iodine: How to Prevent and Survive It.* Victoria, Canada: Trafford Publishing, 2001.

Denning, DW, et al. "Global Burden of Chronic Pulmonary Aspergillosis as Sequel to Pulmonary Tuberculosis." *Bulletin of the World Health Organization* 2011.

Duesberg, PH. "HIV is not the cause of AIDS." *Science* 1988;241:514–517.

Dunn, JT, Delange, F. "Damaged reproduction: the most important consequence of iodine deficiency." *J Clin Endocrinol Metab* 2001;8:2360–63.

Eskin, BA, et al. "Iodine Replacement in Fibrocystic Disease of the Breast." *Can J Surg* 1993;36(5):453–460.

Etzel, R. "Mycotoxins." *JAMA* 2002;287(4).

Fitzpatrick, DQ, Hotz CS, et. al. "Dietary Iodine and Selenium Interact To Affect Thyroid Hormone Metabolism of Rats." *J Nutr* 1997;127(6):1214–1218.

Flechas, Jorge. "Orthoiodosupplementation in a Primary Care Practice." http://www.optimox.com/pics/Iodine/IOD-10/IOD_10.htm.

Francica, JR, et al. "Steric Shielding of Surface Epitopes and Impaired Immune Recognition Induced by the Ebola Virus Glycoprotein." *PLOS Pathogens* 2010;6(9).

Giray, B, et al. "Tissue distribution of Fe, Mn, Cu, and Zn, the essential trace elements associated with oxidant and/or antioxidant processes, was examined in iodine- and/or selenium-deficient rats." *Biol Trace Elem Res* 2003;95(3):247–258.

Guimaraes, MD, et al. "Fungal Infection Mimicking Lung Cancer: A Potential Cause of Misdiagnosis." *Am J Roentgenol* 2013;201(2).

Hamilton, BS. "Influenza Virus-Mediated Membrane Fusion: Determinants of

Hemagglutinin Fusogenic Activity and Experimental Approaches for Assessing Virus Fusion." *Viruses* 2012;4:1144–1168.

Hanahan, D, Weinberg, RA. "The Hallmarks of Cancer." *Cell* 2000;100(1).

Henderson, JN, Tait, IB. "The Use of Povidone-Iodine ('Betadine') Pessaries in the Treatment of Candidal and Trichomonal Vaginitis." *Curr Med Res Opin* 1975;3(3):157–162.

Hodkinson, CF, et al. "Preliminary Evidence of Immune Function Modulation by Thyroid Hormones in Healthy Men and Women Aged 55–70 Years." *J Endocrinol* 2009:55–63.

Hollowell, Joseph, G, et al. "Iodine Nutrition in the United States. Trends and Public Health Implications: Iodine Excretion Data from National Health and Nutrition Examination Surveys I and III (1971–1974 and 1988–1994)." *J Clin Endocrinol Metab* 1998;83(10):3401–3408.

Hsu, Y, Nomura, S. "Sterilization Action of Chlorine and Iodine on Bacteria and Viruses in Water Systems." Baltimore, Maryland: School of Hygiene and Public Health at Johns Hopkins University.

Ichikawa, K. "Induction of cytosolic proteins controlling mitochondrial protein synthesis by thyroid hormone." *J Endocrinol* 1985;61(11):1249–1258.

Institute of Medicine Immunization Safety Review Committee. "Immunization Safety Review: Vaccines and Autism." National Academy of Sciences, 2004.

Institute of Medicine Panel on Micronutrients. *Dietary Reference Intakes for Vitamin A, Vitamin K, Arsenic, Boron, Chromium, Copper, Iodine, Iron, Manganese, Molybdenum, Nickel, Silicon, Vanadium, and Zinc.* Washington, DC: National Academies Press, 2001.

International Medical Veritas Association. "Iodine: Bring Back the Universal Nutrient Medicine." www.health-science-spirit.com/iodine.html.

Jarvis, JC. *Folk Medicine.* New York, NY: Henry Holt & Co., 1958:151.

Java, C, et al. "Evaluation of topical povidone-iodine in chronic suppurative otitis media." *Arch Otolaryngol Head Neck Surg* 2003;129(10):1098–1100.

Kato, Y. "Acidic extracellular microenvironment and cancer." *Cancer Cell International* 2013;13:89.

Kessler, J. "Are there side effects when using supraphysiological levels of iodine in treatment regimens?" *Comprehensive Handbook of Iodine: Nutritional, Endocrine and Pathological Aspects.* San Diego, CA: Academic Press, 2009:801–810.

Kibbler, CC. *Principles and Practice of Clinical Mycology.* Sussex, England: John Wiley and Sons Ltd., 1996.

Küpper, F, et al. "Iodine Uptake in Laminariales involves extracellular, haloperoxidase-mediated oxidation of iodide." *Planta* 1998;207(163).

Langford, WS. *A Comprehensive Guide to Managing Autism.* The Autism File Supplement, 2001.

Lavitelle, D, et al. "Hepatitis C virus glycoproteins mediate low pH-dependent membrane fusion with liposomes." *J Biol Chem* 2006;281(7):3909–3917.

Liu, XY, Jin, TY, Nordberg GF. "Increased urinary calcium and magnesium excretions in rats injected with mercuric chloride." *Pharmacol Toxicol* 1991;68(4):254–259.

The Los Angeles Times. "Research: Staph bug 'steadily growing'" http://www.denverpost.com/breakingnews/ci_7595287.

Madshush, IH, et al. "Mechanism of Entry into the Cytosol of Poliovirus Type 1: Requirement for Low pH." *J Cell Biol* 1984;98:1194–1200.

Maheshwari, RK, et al. "Primary amines enhance the antiviral activity of interferon against a membrane virus: role of intracellular pH." *J Gen Virol* 1991;79:2143–2152.

Marani, L, Venturi, S. "Iodine and Delayed Immunity." *Minerva Med* 1986;77(19):805–809.

Marks, RM, Barton SP, Edwards C. *The Physical Nature of the Skin.* Lancaster: MTP Press, 1988.

Martin, H, Richert, L, Berthelot, Al. "Magnesium Deficiency Induces Apoptosis in Primary Cultures of Rat Hepatocytes." *J Nutr* 2003;133:2505–2511.

Miller, ME, Cappon, CJ. "Anion-Exchange Chromatographic Determination of Bromide in Serum." *Clin Chem* 1984;30(5):781–783.

Miyake, S, et al. "Isotopic Ratio of Radioactive Iodine Released From Fukushima Daiichi NPP Accident." *Geochemical Journal* 2012;46:327–333.

Molnar, I, Magyari, M, Stief, L. "Iodine deficiency in cardiovascular diseases." *Orv Hetil* 1998;139(35):2071–2073.

Murata, A, et al. "Hydroxyl radical as the reactive species in the inactivation of phages by ascorbic acid." *Agric Biol Chem* 1986;50:1481–1487.

National Institutes of Health. "Selenium Fact Sheet." http://ods.od.nih.gov/factsheets/selenium.asp#h5.

Oregon State University. "Iodine." http://lpi.oregonstate.edu/infocenter/minerals/iodine.

Oziol, L, et al. "In vitro free radical scavenging capacity of thyroid hormones and structural analogues." *J Endocrinol* 2001;170:197–206.

Pearce, EN, et al. "Breast Milk Iodine and Perchlorate Concentrations in Lactating Boston-Area Women." *J Clin Endocrin Metab* 2007;92(5):1673–1677.

Pitchford, P. *Healing with Whole Foods, Revised Edition.* Berkeley, CA: North Atlantic Books, 1993.

Potter, S. "Bromine." *A Compend of Materia Medica, Therapeutics, and Prescription Writing.* http://www.henriettesherbal.com/eclectic/potter-comp/bromine.html

Rauws, AG, "Pharmacokinetics of Bromide Ion: An Overview." *Fd Chem Toxic* 1983;21:379–382.

Robey, IF. "Bicarbonate Increases Tumor pH and Inhibits Spontaneous Metastases." *Cancer Res* 2009;68(6).

Rowland, IR, et al. "Effects of diet on mercury metabolism and excretion in mice given methylmercury: role of gut flora." *Arch Environ Health* 1984;39(6).

Saeed, MF, et al. "Cellular Entry of Ebola Virus Involves Uptake by a Macropinocytosis-Like Mechanism and Subsequent Trafficking through Early and Late Endosomes." *PLOS Pathogens* 2010;6(9).

Saker, KE, et al. "Brown seaweed- (Tasco) treated conserved forage enhances antioxidant status and immune function in heat-stressed wether lambs." *J Anim Physiol Anim Nutr* 2004:88:122–130.

Saker, KE, et al. "Tasco-Forage: II. Monocyte immune cell response and performance of beef steers grazing tall fescue treated with a seaweed extract." *J Animal Sci* 2001:79:1022–1031.

Sangster, B, Blom, JL, Sekhuis, VM, et al. "The Influence of Sodium Bromide in Man: A Study in Human Volunteers with Special Emphasis on the Endocrine and the Central Nervous System." *Fd Chem Toxic* 1983;21:409–419.

Schussler, GC, Ranney, HM. "Thyroid Hormones and the Oxygen Affinity of Hemoglobin." *Ann Intern Med* 1971;74:632–633.

Somerset, D, et al. "Differential Expression of JGF and Met in Human Placenta." *J Clin Endocr and Met* 1998;83(4):3401–3408.

Sticht, G, Käferstein, H. "Bromine." *Handbook on Toxicity of Inorganic Compounds.* New York, NY: Marcel Dekker Inc., 1988.

Stoddard, FR, et al. "Iodine alters gene expression in the MCF7 breast cancer cell line: evidence for an anti-estrogen effect of iodine." *Int J Med Sci* 2008;5(4):189–196.

Stone, OJ. "The role of the primitive sea in the natural selection of iodides as a regulating factor in inflammation." *Med Hypotheses* 1988;25:125–129.

Teas, J, et al. "Variability of iodine content in common commercially available edible seaweeds." *Thyroid* 2004;14:836–841.

TEC, Jr. "Paracelsus on What the Physician Should Know." *Pediatrics* 1974;54(2).

Tseng, YL, Latham, KR. "Iodothyronines: oxidative deiodination by hemoglobin and inhibition of lipid peroxidation." *Lipids* 1984;19:96–102.

Turker, O, et al. "Selenium treatment in autoimmune thyroiditis: 9-month follow-up with variable doses." *J Endocrinol* 2006;190(1):151–156.

Vega-Riveroll, L, et al. "Impaired nuclear translocation of estrogen receptor alfa could be associated with the antineoplastic effect of iodine in premenopausal breast cancer." *Cancer Research* 2010;70(24).

Vishniakova, YY, Murav'eva, NI. "On the treatment of dyshormonal hyperplasia of mammary glands." *Vestn Akad Med Nauk SSSR* 1966;21(9):19–22.

Waszkowiak, K, Szymandera-Buszka, K. "Effect of storage conditions on potassium iodide stability in iodized table salt and collagen preparations." *IJFST* 2007;43(5):895–899.

Weill Cornell Medicine Newsroom. "Infections as a Cause of Cancer: A History and Outlook." https://news.weill.cornell.edu/news/2007/12/did-you-know-that-15-to-20-percent-of-cancers-are-caused-by-infections.

Wertenbruch, T, et al. "Serum Selenium levels in patients with remission and relapse of Graves Disease." *Med Chem* 2007;3(3):281–284.

Wesson, LG. *Physiology of the Human Kidney.* New York, NY: Grune and Stratton, 1969: 591.

West, B. "Atrial Fibrillation, Arrhythmias and Iodine." *Health Alert* 2006; 23(6).

Wiles, ME, Wagner, TL, Weglicki, WB. "Effect of acute magnesium deficiency (MgD) on aortic endothelial cell (EC) oxidant production." *Life Sci* 1997;60(3): 221–236.

Winkler, R, Griebenow, S, Wonisch, W. "Effect of iodide on total antioxidant status of human serum." *Cell Biochem Funct* 2000:18:143–146.

Wolff, F. "Transport of iodide and other anions in the thyroid gland." *Physiol Rev* 1964;44:45–90.

Xu, J, et al. "Selenium supplement alleviated the toxic effects of excessive iodine in mice." *Biol Trace Elem Res* 2006;111(1–3):229–238.

Yeargin-Allsopp, M, et al. "Prevalence of autism in a US metropolitan area." *JAMA* 2003; 289: 49–55.

Yun, AJ, et al. "The incorporation of iodine in thyroid hormone may stem from its role as a prehistoric signal of ecologic opportunity: an evolutionary perspective and implications for modern diseases." *Med Hypotheses* 2005;65:804–810.

Zakut, Z, Lotan, M, Bracha, Y. "Vaginal Preparation with Povidone-Iodine before Abdominal Hysterectomy." *Clin Exp Obstet Gynecol* 1987;14(1):1–5.

Zimmermann, MB. "Research on Iodine Deficiency and Goiter in the 19th and Early 20th Centuries." *J Nutr* 2008;138(11):2060–2063.

About the Author

Mark Sircus, Ac., OMD, DM (P), was trained in acupuncture and Asian medicine at the Institute of Traditional Medicine in Santa Fe and the School of Traditional Medicine of New England in Boston. He also served at the Central Public Hospital of Pochutla, Mexico. He is part of the Scientific Advisory and Research Development team of the Da Vinci College of Holistic Medicine. Dr. Sircus' articles have appeared in numerous journals and magazines throughout the world. In addition, he is the best-selling author of several books, including *Sodium Bicarbonate, Healing With Medical Marijuana*, and *Anti-Inflammatory Oxygen Therapy*.

Index

Other Square One Titles of Interest

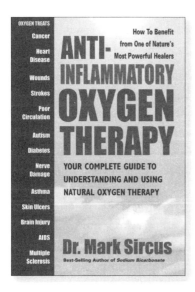

Anti-Inflammatory Oxygen Therapy

Your Complete Guide to Understanding and Using Natural Oxygen Therapy

Dr. Mark Sircus

It is invisible, it is powerful, and it is life sustaining. It is oxygen. We inhale it every day of our lives, and while it makes up only 21 percent of the air we breathe, it is key to our very existence. The more we learn about its healing properties, the more we recognize its tremendous potential as a medical treatment for many serious disorders. Yet few have known about its important therapeutic uses—until now. In his new book, *Anti-Inflammatory Oxygen Therapy,* best-selling author Dr. Mark Sircus examines the remarkable benefits oxygen therapy offers, from detoxification to treatments for a wide variety of disorders—from aging to gastric disorders to cancer.

If you are wondering why you haven't heard about this "miracle" treatment before, the fact is oxygen cannot be patented, it is not expensive, and you don't have to be a specialist to use it. Without a tremendous profit behind it, it's become a well-kept secret, but the facts speak for themselves. In this book, you will learn these life-altering facts—information that could change your health for the better.

$15.95 US • 192 pages • 6 x 9-inch quality paperback • ISBN 978-0-7570-0415-5

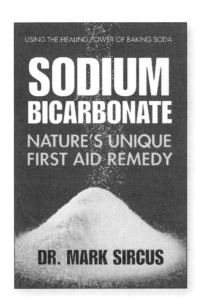

USING THE HEALING POWER OF BAKING SODA

Sodium Bicarbonate

Nature's Unique First Aid Remedy

Dr. Mark Sircus

What if there were a natural health-promoting substance that was inexpensive and available at any grocery store? There is. It's called sodium bicarbonate, also known as baking soda. For years, sodium bicarbonate has been part of a number of hospital treatments, but most people are unaware of its full potential. In this book, Dr. Mark Sircus shows how this compound can be used in the quest for better health.

Sodium Bicarbonate begins with an overview of baking soda, chronicling its use as a home remedy. The author then explains the role sodium bicarbonate plays in pH balance, which is revealed as an important factor in maintaining good health. He then details how this extraordinary substance can alleviate a number of health disorders and suggests the most effective way to use sodium bicarbonate in the treatment of each condition.

More than just a recipe ingredient, baking soda has powerful properties that can allow you to regain your well-being and avoid future health problems. Let *Sodium Bicarbonate* help you look at baking soda in a whole new way.

$16.95 US • 208 pages • 6 x 9-inch paperback • ISBN 978-0-7570-0394-3

Healing with Medical Marijuana

Getting Beyond the Smoke and Mirrors

Dr. Mark Sircus

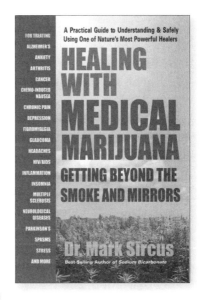

Imagine that there is an effective treatment for dozens of serious ailments—from cancer and Parkinson's disease to headaches and depression. Now imagine that the government is preventing you from using it because it is derived from a controversial herb. Cannabis, more commonly called marijuana, is still looked upon by many people as a social evil; yet, scientific evidence clearly shows that the compounds it contains can reduce, halt, and in many cases, reverse some of our most serious health conditions. In *Healing with Medical Marijuana*, best-selling author and medical researcher Dr. Mark Sircus has written a clear guide to understanding the power of the cannabis plant in combating numerous disorders

While more and more states are now legalizing medical marijuana as a safe and effective treatment method, the controversy continues to block its use for the majority of the population—in spite of the relief it can provide. For those who may be unable to obtain medical marijuana to treat their individual conditions, this book is designed to provide options that can offer the much-needed help they are seeking.

$16.95 US • 192 pages • 6 x 9-inch quality paperback • ISBN 978-0-7570-0441-4

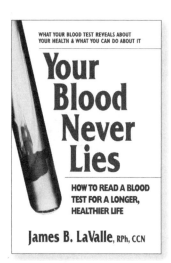

WHAT YOUR BLOOD TEST REVEALS ABOUT
YOUR HEALTH & WHAT YOU CAN DO ABOUT IT

Your Blood Never Lies

HOW TO READ A BLOOD
TEST FOR A LONGER,
HEALTHIER LIFE

James B. LaValle, RPh, CCN

Your Blood Never Lies

How to Read a Blood Test for
a Longer, Healthier Life

James B. LaValle, RPh, CCN

If you're like most people, you probably rely on your doctor to interpret the results of your blood tests, which contain a wealth of information on the state of your health. A blood test can tell you how well your kidneys and liver are functioning, your potential for heart disease and diabetes, the strength of your immune system, the chemical profile of your blood, and many other important facts about the state of your health. And yet, most of us cannot decipher these results ourselves, nor can we even formulate the right questions to ask about them—or we couldn't, until now.

In *Your Blood Never Lies*, best-selling author Dr. James LaValle clears the mystery surrounding blood test results. In simple language, he explains all the information found on a typical lab report—the medical terminology, the numbers and percentages, and the laboratory jargon—and makes it accessible. This means that you will be able to look at your own blood test results and understand the significance of each biological marker being measured. To help you take charge of your health, Dr. LaValle also recommends the most effective standard and complementary treatments for dealing with any problematic findings. Rounding out the book are explanations of lab values that do not appear on the standard blood test, but that should be requested for a more complete picture of your current physiological condition.

Your Blood Never Lies provides the up-to-date information you need to understand your results and take control of your life.

$16.95 US • 368 pages • 6 x 9-inch paperback •
ISBN 978-0-7570-0350-9

Magnificent Magnesium

Your Essential Key to a Healthy Heart & More

Dennis Goodman, MD

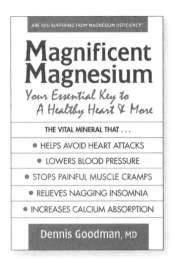

Despite the development of many "breakthrough" drugs designed to combat its effects, heart disease remains the number-one killer of Americans. Is there a simpler solution? The answer is *yes*. For many years, scientists and medical researchers have known about a common mineral that can effectively prevent or remedy many cardiovascular conditions. And unlike the pharmaceuticals usually prescribed, this supplement has no dangerous side effects. In his new book, *Magnificent Magnesium,* world-renowned cardiologist Dr. Dennis Goodman shines a spotlight on magnesium, the mineral that can maximize your heart health.

The author first establishes a firm foundation for understanding heart disease, detailing its many forms and providing a brief overview of its fundamental mechanisms. Next, he examines the important role magnesium plays in many life processes and explore how a deficiency of this substance can lead to many of our nation's most common health conditions, including cardiovascular disease. The author then details magnesium's astounding heart-healthy benefits, along with the additional advantages it provides for other diseases, including obesity, type 2 diabetes, gastrointestinal disorders, osteoporosis, and insomnia. Finally, *Magnificent Magnesium* puts this knowledge to work, offering clear guidelines on how to select and use magnesium supplements to greatest effect.

Many drugs are designed to relieve the symptoms of heart disease, but none of them eliminates the root cause of the problem. In *Magnificent Magnesium,* you will discover how a simple all-natural mineral can improve the function of your heart and help you regain control of your health.

$14.95 US • 192 pages • 6 x 9-inch paperback • ISBN 978-0-7570-0391-2

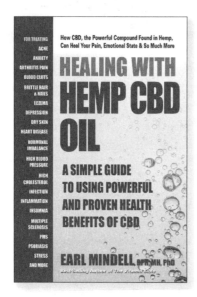

Healing with Hemp CBD Oil

A Simple Guide to Using Powerful and Proven Health Benefits of Hemp

Earl Mindell

The health benefits of marijuana are now getting a good deal of attention. Yet hemp— a close relative of marijuana— is actually a far richer source of CBD, the compound responsible for effectively treating dozens of disorders, and contains very little THC, the substance responsible for marijuana's highs. Sounds like growing and using hemp is a win-win situation, right? Not quite, because the US government, which holds the patent for CBD specifically because of its healing abilities, has unfairly classified hemp as a Class 1 drug, thereby banning people in the United States from growing it commercially. If you find this confusing, you're not alone. That's why best-selling author Earl Mindell has written *Healing with Hemp CBD Oil,* a straightforward book that will first help you understand what's going on with hemp oil in the United States, and then teach you how to use this valuable natural remedy to improve your health.

Although the United States has given CBD-rich hemp a problematic legal status, fortunately, this product—sourced from other countries—is readily available. *Healing with Hemp CBD Oil* guides you in using this all-natural substance as a safe, side effect-free remedy.

$16.95 US • 160 pages • 6 x 9-inch paperback •
ISBN 978-0-7570-0455-1

For more information about our books, visit our website at www.squareonepublishers.com